Infancy: The Basics offers an introduction to the developmental science behind the fascinating world of infant development. This book takes the reader from before birth through the moment infants come into the world seemingly unable to do much but eat, eliminate, and sleep, and across the few short, incredible years, to when infants are walking, talking, thinking humans with clear preferences, wishes, and dreams, having already forged strong long-lasting relationships.

Dispelling common myths and misconceptions about how infants' perception, cognition, language, and personalities develop, this accessible evidence-based book takes a novel whole-child approach and provides insight into the joint roles of nature (biology) and nurture (experience) in infant development, how to care for babies to give them the best start in life, and what it means for infants to become thinking communicating social partners. Topics in this book are covered with an eye firmly fixed on how infants' first years set the stage for the rest of their lives. By helping us understand infants, experts Marc H. Bornstein and Martha E. Arterberry give us the opportunity to learn about the resiliency of our species and the many different contexts in which families rear infants. They cover key topics, including how babies are studied scientifically, prenatal development and the newborn period, how infants explore and understand the world around them, how infants begin to communicate, how infants develop an emotional life, personality, and temperament, how infants build relationships, and how parents succeed in bringing up babies in challenging circumstances.

This concise clear guide to the years from before birth to 3 is for students of developmental psychology, pediatric medicine and nursing, education, and social work. It is also for all parents and professionals caring for infants, who want to understand the secret world of infancy.

Marc H. Bornstein has professional appointments with the Eunice Kennedy Shriver National Institute of Child Health and Human Development (Bethesda), the Institute for Fiscal Studies (London), and UNICEF (NYC). He holds degrees from Columbia College and Yale University as well as Trento and Heidelberg. He edits *Parenting: Science and Practice* and the *Handbook of Parenting*. Bornstein has published in experimental, developmental, and cultural science as well as neuroscience, pediatrics, and aesthetics.

Martha E. Arterberry is the Clara C. Piper Professor of Psychology at Colby College, Maine. She received her B.A. from Pomona College and her Ph.D. from the University of Minnesota. She is the Editor-in-Chief of *Infant Behavior and Development* and Editor of the Lifespan Section of *Acta Psychologica*. Her research focuses on perception, cognition, and action in infancy.

THE BASICS SERIES

The Basics is a highly successful series of accessible guidebooks which provide an overview of the fundamental principles of a subject area in a jargon-free and undaunting format.

Intended for students approaching a subject for the first time, the books both introduce the essentials of a subject and provide an ideal springboard for further study. With over 50 titles spanning subjects from artificial intelligence (AI) to women's studies, *The Basics* is an ideal starting point for students seeking to understand a subject area.

Each text comes with recommendations for further study and gradually introduces the complexities and nuances within a subject.

INFANCY

THE BASICS

**Marc H. Bornstein and
Martha E. Arterberry**

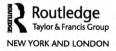

NEW YORK AND LONDON

Cover image: © Getty Images

First published 2023
by Routledge
605 Third Avenue, New York, NY 10158

and by Routledge
4 Park Square, Milton Park, Abingdon, Oxon, OX14 4RN

Routledge is an imprint of the Taylor & Francis Group, an informa business

© 2023 Marc H. Bornstein and Martha E. Arterberry

The right of Marc H. Bornstein and Martha E. Arterberry to be identified as authors of this work has been asserted in accordance with sections 77 and 78 of the Copyright, Designs and Patents Act 1988.

Library of Congress Cataloging-in-Publication Data
Names: Bornstein, Marc H., author. | Arterberry, Martha E., author.
Title: Infancy: the basics / Marc H. Bornstein and Martha E. Arterberry.
Description: New York, NY: Routledge, 2022. |
Includes bibliographical references and index.
Identifiers: LCCN 2021062681 (print) | LCCN 2021062682 (ebook) |
ISBN 9781032001142 (hardback) | ISBN 9781032001159 (paperback) |
ISBN 9781003172802 (ebook)
Subjects: LCSH: Infant psychology. | Infants—Development.
Classification: LCC BF719 .B67 2022 (print) | LCC BF719 (ebook) |
DDC 155.42/2—dc23/eng/20220111
LC record available at https://lccn.loc.gov/2021062681
LC ebook record available at https://lccn.loc.gov/2021062682

ISBN: 978-1-032-00114-2 (hbk)
ISBN: 978-1-032-00115-9 (pbk)
ISBN: 978-1-003-17280-2 (ebk)

DOI: 10.4324/9781003172802

Typeset in Palatino
by codeMantra

Dedication (MHB)
For Lewis

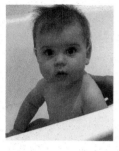

This *Basics Book* about **Infancy** advances a "whole child" perspective on the beginnings of life.

Although individual chapters treat infancy in terms of growing, thinking, communicating, feeling, and relating, in reality all these remarkable achievements of the opening years are ineluctably bound together. In evidence, consider one fleeting moment in the life of an 8-month-old as it attests to the inextricability of perception-action-thought-emotion-relation.

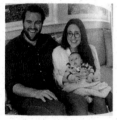

Propped in the crook of a couch, Lewis was being read some baby books. After three or so, next up was a picture book constructed wholly of photos from Lewis's first 6 months. When the page was turned to this picture of Lewis himself sitting with his parents, Lewis spontaneously and promptly leaned forward and kissed his mother's face:

perception-action-thought-emotion-relation.

In Memoriam (MEA)
For Brooke (2000–2019)

Whose all-too-brief life illuminated the marvels of development and what can be accomplished by human perseverance.

CONTENTS

ILLUSTRATIONS

TABLES

PREFACE

This is a book about infancy, arguably the third stage of life. The *third* stage? Well, infants come into the world after about 40 weeks of gestation, meaning the second stage of human life is the approximate 9 prenatal months that take place after conception and before birth. The *second* stage? Scientists have come to understand on many grounds that the health, knowledge, and behavior of parents-to-be and their parents going back untold numbers of generations help to shape the future well-being of the infant, and so in a real sense constitute the first stage of life. That is, the many decisions and actions of our forebears in a meaningful degree chart our path. Indeed, the only reason you are reading this book is that each one of your ancestors going back into the mists of time succeeded in living and reproducing. So, yes, infancy – the subject of this book – is the *third* stage of human development.

Why does the world need another book about babies? Indeed, why have we written this book at all? Why have philosophers, psychologists, and physicians paid so much attention to infants and infancy? Infants instill curiosity in everyone who comes into contact with them, and people, parents, and professionals of many stripes are captivated by infancy for many reasons. First, infancy offers the opportunity for us to come to know things about ourselves from when we started out in life. People are simultaneously similar and different. When do individual differences begin, and what are their origins? How does that variation reflect the genetic endowment of parents, and how does experience get under the skin? Second, parents are interested and invested in practical matters of infant survival, socialization, and education. The pervasiveness, rapidity, and clarity of development in infancy make this stage of life fascinating. We witness seemingly daily changes in the shape and capacity of the baby's body as well as the growth of the baby's sensory and perceptual capacities, the baby's abilities to make sense of and master things in the world, eventually to achieve communication, to gain a personality, and to forge social bonds. Today's new moms and dads also know that the brain that underpins all these developments, like the major part of an iceberg hidden from view, is fast maturing itself. Finally, politicians and policymakers are (or should be!) interested in infants because their well-being represents investment in the next generation and in the success of society itself. Interventions that start early and target socioemotional and cognitive skill building and provide family support result in higher graduation rates, lower rates of teen pregnancy, better salaries, and reduced reliance on public assistance. In terms of economies of investment, optimizing early child development provides a better rate of return than programs targeting and attempting to remediate later periods in the lifespan. These are some of the reasons why we have written a whole book about this relatively brief but formative period of the life course.

An additional reason is the unique approach to infancy this book takes. *Infancy: The Basics* is about babyhood but is not a pediatric compendium of medical diagnosis and treatment. Nor is it an opinion vent on breast-vs.-bottle or an operating "how-to" manual to put a baby down to sleep, etc. Rather, *Infancy: The Basics* conveys hard-won knowledge about infancy from developmental science and is premised on the belief that, knowing more about development in infancy, today's and tomorrow's parents will make better informed decisions about how to care for and interact with their precious little ones.

Developmental science is an evidence-based empirical approach to the lifespan study of human growth, maturation, and experience. So, developmental science is concerned with infants' feeding, crying, and sleeping (traditional interests of new parenthood)... but so much more. The topics of developmental science that are germane to infancy are health and physical growth, mental and verbal growth, and emotional and social growth. These are the topics of the chapters that follow, and we distill "the basics" – the important lessons from the innumerable scientific publications on infancy written by professionals of all stripes – from anthropologists to zoologists. Through close research, developmental scientists answer questions about what babies see and hear, think and understand, feel and do. Why and how babies develop. *Infancy: The Basics* recounts what developmental scientists have learned about the majesty and mystery of infancy.

Marc H. Bornstein
Martha E. Arterberry

INFANCY: THE BASICS – HOW HAVE ITS CHAPTERS BEEN ORGANIZED?

Chapter 1 Infancy raises five questions about infancy, answers to which inform all later chapters on substantive topics of infant development. What are the principal topics with which the developmental science of infancy studies is concerned? What drives infant development – biology? experience? or the two together? Is infancy important to the rest of life? What is the "whole child" view of infancy? How have infants revealed secrets about themselves and their development? The substantive chapters that build on answers to these five questions concern growing, thinking, communicating, feeling, and relating.

Chapter 2 Growing looks at topics of genetics, nervous system function, and physical development in infancy as important issues in themselves and explores how they pave the path to development in thinking, communicating, feeling, and relating. Insights from genetics, anatomy, and birth provide a deeper understanding of infants' earliest capacities.

Chapter 3 Thinking describes some of the main ways developmental scientists have concluded that infants perceive and learn and determined how infants remember as well as what infants do with the knowledge they accrue. Faithful to the whole-child view, infants apply all sorts of thinking to communicating, feeling, and relating.

Chapter 4 Communicating first defines broad domains of language, issues of norms and individual variation, as well as methods of infant language study and then describes how infants develop from speechless individualists into interactive conversationalists, ready and able to articulate their cares, needs, and desires to others as well as the many supports parents provide infants on their way to acquiring language.

Chapter 5 Feeling treats infants' expressions and perceptions of primary and secondary emotions, infants' different styles of temperament, and the route to the development of a self in infancy.

Chapter 6 Relating recounts the many sophisticated capacities infants bring to establishing relationships with significant others in their lives as well as influences on infant relationships that are proximal to the infant, like parents and the infant's local environment, and more distal systems of influence in social class, ethnicity, culture, and time.

Chapter 7 Coda; Appreciating the Whole Child uses the development of social cognition in infancy – the ways that infants perceive and understand their interactions with other people, come to know and rely on people with whom they interact, and appreciate differences between their own perspectives and knowledge and those of others – to bring home the idea that growing, thinking, communicating, feeling, and relating in infants are intimately integrated and mutually reinforcing domains of chilkd development.

ACKNOWLEDGMENTS

We thank the infants and parents who have voluntarily participated in developmental science over the last half century and con-
tributed to the corpus of knowledge that made this book possible.
We also thank E. Chung, C. Hurson, T. Montgomery, Y. Tojoula,
and A. A. D. Vieux for help preparing this work. Finally, we thank
H. Pritt and the team at Routledge/Taylor & Francis for affording
us the opportunity to contribute to The Basics series and for their
helpful guidance throughout.

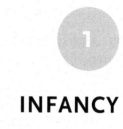

INFANCY

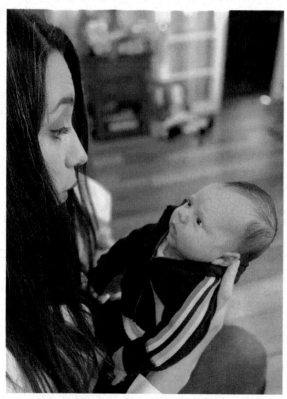

(Courtesy of M. H. Bornstein).

DOI: 10.4324/9781003172802-1

INTRODUCTION

By definition, infancy is the period of life between birth and the emergence of language roughly one and one-half to two years later. Infancy thus encompasses only a small fraction of the average person's life expectancy, and readers may therefore wonder why we have written a whole book about so brief a period of the lifespan, and why philosophers, psychologists, and physicians have paid so much attention to infancy. Three broad reasons traditionally answer that curiosity and motivate studying infancy scientifically: They are philosophical and scientific questions, parental investment, and applied concerns. To them, we add a fourth reason: Infants are fascinating, and we hope you will agree with the value of all four by the time you conclude reading this book.

Infants rely on others to meet all their survival, mental, social, and emotional needs. The very word *infancy* derives from what must be the most salient characteristic of the first year or so of life, infants' inability to speak (the Latin *in+fans*, literally means "nonspeaker"). Infants cannot even make their state and basic needs (never mind their wishes and dreams) clearly known to their caregivers. Parents are faced moment-to-moment with trying to understand and respond to each cry or vocalization. Is that cry *I want to eat, I want to sleep, I want to be held,* or *I want to play*? For parents, meeting their infants' needs can be exhilarating when they are successful and excruciating when they fail. For their part, infants find themselves wanting something – to eat or sleep, to be held or play – without being able simply to say so. Saving the day, even within this nonverbal period, infants develop many ways to help their parents understand and respond appropriately to their needs.

In spite of its brevity, development in infancy is dramatic *and* fast. For infants' parents, the days are long, but the years are short, so that before they know it the toddler is emerging from the infant (and, all too soon after, the child from the toddler). The rapidity of development in every sphere of the infant's life – from breastfeeding to the introduction of solids, from sleeping at any moment to settling into a schedule, from disorganized arm and leg movements to intentional reaching and walking, from vegetative vocalizations to syllables and words – rivets and fascinates watchful parents.

In this chapter, we raise five questions about infancy, answers to which inform all later chapters on substantive topics of infant development. The substantive chapters in this book that answer these five questions concern growing, thinking, communicating, feeling, and relating.

1. What are the principal topics in infancy science?
2. What drives infant development – biology? experience? or the two together? A perennial concern of infancy is the relative contributions of "nature" (biology) and "nurture" (experience) to early development. How much of what a baby is (and eventually who we are) reflects genetic inheritance from parents, and how much the experiences parents provide infants? More to the point, how do these two life forces complement one another?
3. Is infancy important to the rest of life? Infancy could be the initial phase of a seamless or continuous lifeline in that who infants are and what they experience connect to and foretell child, adolescent, or even adult development. Or, infancy could be a separate stage of the life cycle and discontinuous with child, adolescent, and adult development. (See Box 1.1 for more on this question.)
4. What is the whole-child view of infancy? Contemporary developmental science research has now revealed a goodly amount about infants and their development. Historically that information was acquired piecemeal: Developmental scientists focused on perception or cognition or emotion. However, in real life all the parts of infants work together, and *whole is greater than the sum of its parts*. This book treats infants' growing, thinking, communicating, feeling, and relating through the lens of the "whole child."
5. How do infants reveal secrets about themselves and their development? The chapters in this book concentrate on the *whats*, *hows*, and *whys* of specific areas of infant development. The story would be far from complete, however, without describing the ways developmental scientists have achieved an understanding of infancy. Thus, we also address how we know what babies know and can do based on the methods of developmental science.

This chapter introduces major theoretical underpinnings, burning questions, and research procedures that have been leveraged by developmental scientists to gain the knowledge that is conveyed in substantive chapters about infancy that follow. We begin by briefly answering the first question: What are the principal topics in infancy science?

BOX 1.1   Stages of Life

Many laypeople and some developmental scientists divide the lifespan into easy-to-understand stages: infancy, childhood, adolescence, adulthood, and old age. A stage is commonly defined as a complex pattern of interrelated features. However, not all developmental scientists think this way or even believe in stages at all. On the one hand, dividing the life cycle into identifiable stages seems intuitive, and self-evident physical, motor, verbal, and cognitive components of development support this viewpoint. Infants creep and crawl, whereas children walk and run; infants do not speak, whereas children do. Many generally well-known developmental theorists – Freud, Piaget, and Erikson – championed stage theories of development. On the other hand, alternative views assert that development unfolds as a series of gradual transitions. James (1890, p. 237) wrote that development is *without break, crack, or division.* Infants at first on their backs wave their legs about (hopefully a lot of the time in the "happy baby" yoga position), then when they flip over eventually rock on all fours, then they might move about on their backs or rumps, then creep, then standing and cruising around holding on to coffee table sides, then toddle, a bit, then begin to walk more steadily on two feet, mixing up these accomplishments from time to time. The same goes for talking: Vegetative sounds turn into cooing and babbling and then rudimentary syllables and then real words and so forth. Moreover, even structures and functions in infants that appear to undergo discrete stage-like changes absorb and build on prior achievements. The characteristics of one stage might distinguish it from preceding and succeeding stages; yet the accomplishments of earlier stages are carried into and mesh with new elements that anticipate later ones. Stages are problematic because they oversimplify development and downplay differences and variation: Stages are general and idealistic, but life is filled with nuance and inconsistency. Stage theories of development smack of a belief in biological maturation as the dominant force guiding development, and they are unidirectional in time, irreversible in sequence, universal, and goal directed. However, development does not always (or necessarily) entail progression toward a given end. For developmental scientists, a key question is whether humans develop in the way an acorn grows into an oak (through incremental and continuous change) or as a caterpillar becomes a butterfly (through dramatic and discontinuous change)? The answer (as in most of science) is, it "depends ...."

PRINCIPAL TOPICS OF INFANCY STUDIES

At its most basic level, developmental science is concerned, first, with describing and understanding the status of different **structures** of the developing human (for example, the visual or auditory systems of the brain) and their **functions** (for example, seeing and hearing). Second, developmental scientists focus on questions of structure and function at different points early in life to address questions about the **origins** of different structures and functions and how those structures and functions **develop**. So, for example, with regard to speech, infants begin life uttering only vegetative sounds, like grunts and cries, to communicate their needs, like hunger. By the end of infancy, the child is using simple language to function in the same way, "more milk." Similarly, with regard to motor function, young infants start out exploring features of objects by mouthing them. As their motor skills improve, they coordinate their hands, fingers, and eyes to gain more advanced information.

BIOLOGY? EXPERIENCE? OR THE TWO TOGETHER?

What makes the structures and functions in infants what they are, and what forces guide their development? When do structures and functions emerge, and why and how do they change with age (if at all)? Is development biologically programmed (nature) or guided by experience (nurture)? The earliest interest in these questions was expressed by philosophers and clergy who chose clear sides. It was either biology *or* experience, nature *or* nurture. These questions were answered by so-called **nativists** who argued that mental and moral life are instinctive or inborn and by so-called **empiricists** who argued that knowledge and ethics are products of experience in the world.

Today we are amused to realize that many of the greatest philosophical and religious thinkers of the past were so occupied with the minds and morals of *babies*. It is nonetheless true. Philosophy and religion alike long obsessed with where our intelligence and scruples come from and how they might develop (or be developed) over time. Are good and evil inborn or are they learned?

The British philosopher John Locke (1632–1704) exemplifies the empiricist school of thought. Locke asserted that human beings possess no knowledge of the world when they are born. He famously described the infant mind as a *tabula rasa* or "blank slate." Instead, Locke contended that mental and moral development reflect what we experience and learn as we grow. Even passing familiarity with a 1-month-old might convince a parent observer that, indeed, this *fetus ex utero* (fetus outside the uterus) knows pretty much nothing. The U.S. philosopher William James (1842–1910) advanced a slightly different empiricist view, namely that the world of the infant is a *blooming, buzzing confusion*. There might be something in the infant mind, but it is definitely a jumble. In James's view, development consists less of acquiring knowledge and more of accruing experiences that organize the mind to create order. From this empiricist view, infants are innocent and naive and develop into cognitively and socially thoughtful and ethical mature adults.

By contrast, philosophers in the nativist school decried the empiricist assertion – that human beings begin life empty headed – as both morally intolerable and logically indefensible. On Biblical interpretation, God would not create mindless creatures "in His image." They also asserted that good or evil must be inborn because neither could be learned in the course of a short childhood. The French philosopher René Descartes (1596–1650) exemplifies this nativist point of view. He proposed that even young infants are born with ideas which start them off in understanding the world and that the human mind imposes order on experience from the environment. Other philosophers like the English Thomas Hobbes (1588–1679) and the Swiss Jean-Jacques Rousseau (1712–1778) were nativists but came down on the opposing sides of the question of infant innocence: for Rousseau the human "state of nature" is innocent and good, without envy, distrust, or conflict, and is perfectible, whereas for Hobbes the *life of man [is] solitary, poor, nasty, brutish, and short.*

In its extreme form, nativists believed that, if the infant's heredity is good, then the infant's development and maturity will be good, regardless of whether the infant's environment or experiences are good or bad. Similarly, if the infant's heredity is bad, then the infant's development and maturity will be bad, regardless of whether the infant's environment or experiences are bad or good. By contrast, nurturists predicted that, if the infant's environment or experiences are good, then the infant's development and maturity will be good, regardless of the infant's heredity. And, if the infant's environment or experiences are bad, then the infant's development and maturity will bad, regardless of heredity.

Nativism and empiricism did not die in the past, but both lived on well into the 20th century with advocates still active in the 21st century. For example, the U.S. psychologist John B. Watson (1878–1958) famously declared for empiricism:

> *Give me a dozen healthy infants, well-formed, and my own specified world to bring them up in, and I'll guarantee to take any one at random and train him to become any type of specialist I might select—doctor, lawyer, artist, merchant-chief and yes, even beggarman and thief, regardless of his talents, penchants, tendencies, abilities, vocations, race of his ancestors.*
>
> (Watson, 1924, p. 104)

In stark contrast, the U. S. pediatrician Arnold Gesell (1880–1961), who was "America's Baby Doctor" before the Second World War (and a contemporary of Watson), wrote forcefully in support of nativism that *the original impulse to growth... is endogenous rather than exogenous* (1924, p. 354) meaning that forces internal to the child drive development and not experiences external to the child. Many of today's dyed-in-the-wool geneticists are likewise nativists who diagnose and treat mental illness, cancer, and other human afflictions as pure products of biology with little or no regard for the environments, life experiences, and behaviors of people that may give rise to disease.

In the years since philosophical and spiritual opinions dominated, scientific researchers have attempted to parse the contributions of nature and nurture to infancy and infant development, often relying on what are called **natural experiments**. For example, researchers can compare identical (monozygotic or MZ) twins, who share 100% of their genes, with fraternal (dizygotic or DZ) twins, who share only 50% of their genes, but who as siblings born at the same time and growing in the same family share the same environment. If heredity prevails, MZ twins should be more alike than DZ twins on a particular characteristic. Similarly, MZ twins reared in different families can be compared with MZ twins reared in the same family to determine the effect of varying experience for a presumably genetically identical characteristic. One such study looked at the heritability of dyslexia by comparing its co-occurrence in MZ twins (68%) versus DZ twins (38%; DeFries et al., 1987). These kinds of results point to a genetic component to dyslexia, but it is important to note that concordance between MZ twins is almost never 100%, indicating that experience also plays a role and whether co-occurrence in MZ twins is even greater than co-occurrence in DZ twins depends on the structure or function. Other natural experiments compare biological children and adoptive children being reared in the same family. Biological children share genes with their parents, whereas adoptive children do not. So, if intelligence or personality is inherited, biological children should be more like their parents than are adopted children.

Natural experiments are just that, natural, and so they are not properly controlled experiments. It is not possible in an experiment of nature to scientifically manipulate all variables. For example, it is possible that some parents would treat MZ twins similarly and DZ twins differently, so that MZ twins turn out to be more alike than DZ twins not because of genetics but because of experience.

With advances in mapping the human genome, researchers are empowered with new tools to unravel more realistically how interactions between genetic makeup and environmental experiences affect infants and the course of development. One such study identified a particular gene variant in children with Attention Deficit and Hyperactivity Disorder (ADHD) and high novelty seeking (Qian et al., 2018). These same children also seem to be more responsive to the environments in which they are born, that is they respond more strongly to low- and high-quality parenting than children without that genetic variant. Those children with the gene variant common to ADHD may be more distractible and less able to concentrate to learn things about the world, but because they are also responsive to high-quality parenting, patient parenting can effectively help offset their otherwise detrimental ADHD tendencies. **Epigenetics** is the modern study of how experience and environment affect when and how genes express themselves. Two people may have the same gene, but their different experiences can alter how that gene works. Moreover, this interaction begins during pregnancy; prenatal adaptations to the uterine environment prepare the fetus for post-natal life (Camerota & Willoughby, 2021). In short, genetics and experiences codetermine development. MZ twins who (are thought to) share 100% of their genes are never identical – even at birth. MZ twins experience different environments with respect to many characteristics even during gestation in the uterus before birth; access to nutrition or different opportunities to move are examples. Figure 1.1 shows genetically identical littermate rodents exposed to different *in utero* and post-natal experiences.

Questions about nature and nurture are not solely theoretical and without practical implications. Which theory one subscribes to has real-world consequences. If you (or society) believe that intelligence or personality is fixed by genetics, then you (and society) are unlikely to provide experiences that foster greater intelligence or personality adjustment in children. Why bother? Genes make all the difference, and experience will have little or no effect. If, however, you believe that experiences are determinative of intelligence or personality in children, it is incumbent on you (and society) to provide children with the experiences children need to develop optimally.

Most contemporary developmental scientists no longer subscribe to pure empiricism or pure nativism, but rather favor a **transactional model** of development. This approach contends that the organism and the environment, genes and experience, the infant and the parent mutually influence one another over time. That is, nature and nurture work together to shape infant development in dynamic,

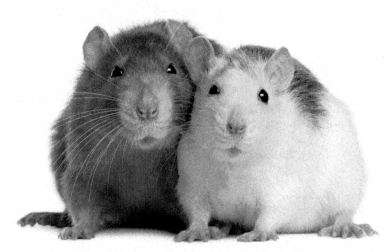

Figure 1.1 Different *in utero* experiences alter the expression of genes (DNA) which results in different organisms even with identical genetic make-up.

interactive, evolving ways. An important feature of transaction is that individuals help to plot the course of their own development. Figure 1.2 portrays the transaction between the infant and a parent through time. Infants' characteristics influence the experiences they are exposed to, how they interpret those experiences, and the ways those experiences affect them, which ultimately influences infant development. As can be seen in Figure 1.2, the infant (I) at Time 1 (T1) influences the parent (P) at Time 2 (T2) who influences the infant (I) at Time 3 (T3). For example, a hungry crying baby cues the mother to feed the baby, which permits the now sated baby to explore and learn from the environment and to engage more with mother. Figure 1.2 shows three general sources of infant development. Infants contribute directly to their own development; infants contribute indirectly to their development by the influence they exert on their parents; and parents contribute directly to infants' development.

The infant's experience and effective environment are not limited to the infant's immediate surroundings. The effective environment includes peers, schools, social networks, communities, and culture. The U.S.-Russian developmental scientist Urie Bronfenbrenner (1917–2005) proposed a **Bioecological Systems Theory** that captures the roles of environment and experience in child development (Figure 1.3). The infant is embedded in a system of nested

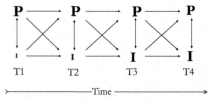

Figure 1.2 In the transactional model, the Infant (I) grows and changes and the Parent (P) changes over time as each also influences the other in a continual process of development and change. (Created by M. H. Bornstein, after Bornstein, 2009.)

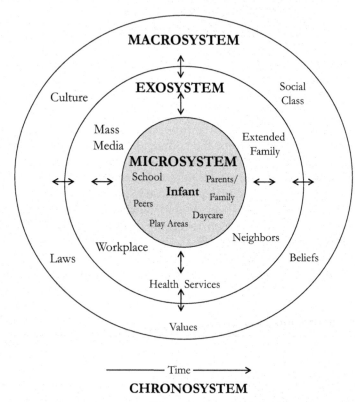

Figure 1.3 Adapted after the Bioecological Systems Theory of development. (Created by M. H. Bornstein.)

environments and experiences that resemble Russian nested dolls. Some environments and experiences are in close and constant proximity to the infant during development (parents and toys, for example); other environments and experiences are increasingly distant from the infant but are still influential in the infant's development (neighbors, mass media, and cultural beliefs, for example).

The timing of experiences can be determinative in infancy in addition to the way experiences shape early development. Developmental science has identified three temporal models of when experiences can affect development. In one model, an experience uniquely affects the infant at one early time and the effect of that early experience continues independent of other later experiences. Babies who grow up in Chicago learn to speak English, and even if they move to Paris later in life they continue to be able to speak English. In a second model, an early experience may have no effect on the infant at the time, but that experience uniquely affects the infant at a later time point. Early good nutrition is known to affect growth at puberty in adolescence. These first two models operate through **sensitive periods**, that is experiences at specific times exert lasting short- or long-term effects (see Box 1.2). In a third model, a given experience influences development because it persists and so cumulates in its impact. Persistent poverty piles up from infancy through childhood to erode adult mental health.

Neither biological predispositions nor environmental experiences alone determine the beginning, direction, end, or final resting level of development. Rather, these life forces continuously influence one another in development. Today, infancy researchers are interested in learning which experiences affect what aspects of development when and how, the ways in which individual children with their particular biological endowments are so affected, as well as the ways in which individual children affect their own development.

The fact that infants are genetically constituted in unique ways combined with the fact that each infant encounters unique experiences in growing up means that the paths along which infants develop are unique and result in all the wonderful individual differences that make up humanity. In a given year, approximately 4 million new babies are born in the United States. The wonder is that for the 11,000 babies born every day, a number equivalent to the population of a small town, each one is exceptional and special. Different people naturally understand the world in unique ways because of their unique genetic and experiential histories. As the U.S. writer and literary critic Edmund Wilson (1895–1972) noted, *no two persons ever read the same book* (Wilson, 1948). In developmental science

BOX 1.2   Set for Life? A Natural Experiment

How do we know whether experiences in infancy relate to later in life? One way is to look at natural experiments, such as The Bucharest Early Intervention Project. A group of investigators took advantage of orphanage practices in Romania to study the effects of extreme deprivation and intervention on infant and child development. At the time the study began, the Romanian state cared for all orphaned children in institutions. During the course of the study, half of the children remained in an institution, and the other half went to live with foster families. The children varied in age when they were placed in foster care, and the researchers grouped them as placed before 24 months or after 24 months of age. In addition, another group of families with same-aged children served as a never-institutionalized control (because they were not orphans). By studying these children longitudinally, the researchers determined which developmental processes were permanently affected by early deprivation and which were not. For example, children who experienced institutional care and foster care had lower IQ scores at age 8 years than those who were never in institutional care. Moreover, children who were institutionalized, regardless of foster care placement or not, did not respond to stressful situations in the same way as never-institutionalized children (McLaughlin et al., 2015). This natural experiment provides us with important information about early development. The researchers found compromises in nearly every aspect of development among the institutional group, and the effect of foster care placement, especially before 24 months, attenuated the effects of early deprivation in some domains of child development. These findings suggest that it is "easier and more efficient to build a 'brain' correctly the first time than it is to rebuild it following injury and adversity" (Nelson et al., 2014, p. 322).

terms, as individual biology and experience aggregate in life, the result is increasing individual specificity.

IS INFANCY IMPORTANT?

The significance of infancy and development in infancy has also been debated by two extreme schools of thought. One school believes that infancy is not really all that important because the status of the infant or experiences in infancy have little (if any) long-term or predictive significance. Whatever early developments may occur, they can be altered after infancy. Another school argues that development in infancy is important in itself and for later life. For these theorists, social orientations, motivations, and intellectual predilections established in infancy set lifelong patterns. Once again, too, which side of the argument you (or society) comes down on has telling implications. If you (or society) believe that infancy is a passing phase without long-term meaning, then do not worry about babies and do not waste investments on infant toys or enrichment programs. If, however, you (or society) believe that infancy is a phase of life that is important and prognostic of later development, then by all means invest in infant care and nurturance, sociality and education. The benefit to society depends on it.

Who were prominent proponents of the importance of infancy and infant experience, and why did they believe what they did? Philosophers of many persuasions as far back in time as Plato (*ca.* 350 BCE), and scientists from biology and embryology to neuroscience and psychology, have considered infancy to be uniquely important for several reasons:

1.   The immature nervous system is especially plastic to experience
2.   Neoteny, the prolongation of infancy especially in human beings, allows the developing organism time to adapt to the environment
3.   What is experienced or learned first has lasting influences
4.   Infants have an extraordinary facility for learning

All of these facts imply that early experiences exert an outsized effect the course of subsequent development.

The line-up of world-renowned proponents of the importance of infancy is impressive. Sigmund Freud (1856–1939), the Austrian neurologist and the founder of psychoanalysis, first focused attention on infancy, asserting that the ways babies are treated establish their lifelong personality traits. Later Erik Erikson (1902–1994), the U.S.-German developmental psychologist and psychoanalyst, contended that experiences in infancy of trust or mistrust set the person down one or another lifelong path. Likewise, behaviorists and learning theorists like Watson and B. F. Skinner (1904–1990), the U.S. psychologist, stressed the importance of infant experiences because they occur first, have no competing propensities to replace, and thus facilitate rapid learning. Ethological researchers of animal behavior, like the Austrian Konrad Lorenz (1903–1989) and the Dutchman Niko Tinbergen (1907–1988), and embryological researchers of prenatal physiology, like the U.S. Gilbert Gottlieb (1929–2006), all emphasized the special role of early experiences in terms of sensitive periods. Additional evidence for the importance of infancy was offered by Jean Piaget (1896–1980), the Swiss psychologist who theorized that higher-order intellectual capacities build on simpler early developments. Similarly, early biological and behavioral patterns (like temperament) are believed to underlie more complex behavioral patterns (like personality traits). Modern attachment theorists, like the British psychoanalyst John Bowlby (1907–1990) and the U.S.-Canadian developmental scientist Mary Ainsworth (1913–1999), as well as language theorists, like the U.S linguist Eric Lenneberg (1921–1975), equally assigned great importance to emotional and verbal experiences that occur in infancy and likely have long-lasting influences.

Other research has failed to support the importance of infancy and undermined confidence in the belief that infancy or early experiences have consequential influences. Some theorists have argued that experiences in infancy are peripheral or ephemeral, in the sense that they are fleeting and have little or no enduring effects. Gesell, for example, concluded that, like anatomy, the psychology of the individual unfolds on the basis of a maturing biological program that is largely unaffected by experience. The U.S. developmental scientist Jerome Kagan (1929–2021) pointed to research indicating that major differences in infants' rearing environments – from daycare to culture – have little apparent effect on the way children basically develop. Furthermore, many interventions beginning in infancy have not always succeeded in demonstrating long-term rewards, and critics like the U.S. educational psychologist Arthur Jensen (1923–2012) used such findings to argue that early interventions may be wasteful. Finally, time and again human beings have proved resilient and able to recover from deprivations of various sorts, undermining the view that early experience is determinative of outcomes in life.

As with the nature/nurture debate, the truth is likely "it depends…". For example, the significance of infancy as a stage in life could vary with different structures or functions. Even if later developments replace statuses in infancy, one cannot observe a baby from birth to 18 months without being amazed at the growth taking place before one's eyes. By the end of infancy, a child has learned the basics of language, how to walk, how to eat, to recognize and bond with caregivers, the basics of cause and effect, the physics of how people and things move and act on each other, and the list goes on. These accomplishments of infancy are either lifelong achievements in themselves or the elements of lifelong achievements. On these grounds, we think infancy is important.

THE WHOLE-CHILD VIEW OF INFANCY

Both authors of this book have taught college-level courses on infancy. When confronted with the goal of organizing the increasingly vast amount of information about infants and conveying a sense of the infant child, the would-be teacher must make a fundamental decision. Do I organize the information by age? If yes, the lectures and readings would unfold like this: 1-month-olds are so and so physically developed, perceive the world in such and such a way, are capable of this or that kind of thinking, display one but not another kind of emotion, and so forth for 2-month-olds, for 3-month-olds, and on and on to the end of infancy. This approach would certainly paint a rich picture of infants at each age, but would convey only a lurching sense of how physical growth, perception, cognition, and emotions each develops dynamically over infancy. This is the so-called **chronological** approach. The alternative approach is to track physical, perceptual, cognitive, emotional, and social development dynamically as each unfolds over the course of infancy. This is the so-called **topical** approach, and the approach we take in this book. Each approach has advantages and disadvantages, but one must choose.

It was the case not long ago, and still is for reasons to be explained shortly, that individual researchers in infancy focus on one or another structure or function of infant development – physical growth, perception, emotions, and so forth – often to the exclusion of others. Most did so at a single time point in infancy to describe structure or function. Some studied the topic in the same babies across time (a **longitudinal design**) or different-aged babies at the same time (**cross-sectional design**; see Box 1.3). Practically speaking, it is difficult enough to study (and to speak about) just one structure or function at one age let alone multiple structures or functions across ages. However, this narrow approach short-changes infants.

In response, developmental scientists now acknowledge the deeper reality of a systems perspective on infant development. Development in the systems perspective is dynamic in the sense that the organization of the infant system as a whole reflects the activity of all the infants' different structures and functions as each and all change as the infant matures and gains new experiences. So, as any one infant system emerges (for example, a change in physical growth like the change from crawling to standing upright and cruising and walking), that emergence and change bring a host of new experiences that influence and are influenced by the emergence and changes in related component systems (so the newly standing infant sees the world much differently from the infant who is confined to crawling). Thus, development is dynamic and systemic, taking place across different systems at the same time. Walking has major implications for both cognitive and social development.

BOX 1.3   Two Developmental Principles and Two Developmental Research Designs

Central to questions of the long-term significance of infancy is the extent to which a structure or function is consistent over time.

1. **Stability** describes consistency over time in the relative standing of individuals in a group on some structure or function in development. For example, activity level in infants would be stable if some infants are more active than others when they are young and they continue to be more active than others when they are older. Stability is concerned with individual differences.

2. **Continuity** describes consistency over time in a group on some structure or function in development. For example, activity level would be continuous if as a group, infants are as active on average when they are young as when they are older. Continuity is concerned with group mean level.

Thus, a structure or function can be developmentally stable and continuous, stable and discontinuous, unstable and continuous, or unstable and discontinuous.

Central to determining the extent to which a structure or function is consistent over time is the developmental design used to study the structure or function. Two main research designs have been adopted to address questions of consistency. Each has advantages and disadvantages.

1. **Longitudinal** designs involve repeated measurement of the same infants over time and constitute a principal method for assessing development. The longitudinal design provides the only means of evaluating stability or continuity in the same infants. However, longitudinal studies are costly, take a long time to complete, and not all infants are always available for testing at every age.

2. **Cross-sectional** designs compare different groups of infants of different ages. Cross-sectional designs can be completed in shorter amounts of time than longitudinal designs (researchers do not have to wait for the babies to grow up), but cross-sectional designs do not allow developmental assessment of stability of individual differences within the same babies.

Infants' interactions with both people and objects change once they can move about, no longer confining the use of their hands to crawling. Before standing upright, infants view the world from lying positions or from 6 to 8 inches (15–20 cm) above the ground while sitting or crawling. Suddenly, cruising or toddling babies can view the world from a height of 2 feet (30.5 cm), and a whole new array of objects can be approached, explored, manipulated, and mastered. These new experiences, in turn, push cognitive and socioemotional development. After being wholly dependent on adults for stimulation, toddlers can now rapidly acquire abilities to explore and to discover stimulation independently. As far as socioemotional development is concerned, the ability to stand instigates significant changes of different sorts in the infants' role vis-á-vis adults. In addition to exploring their environment, infants now have control over their proximity to other people, and so they can approach or withdraw at will. They can examine objects (like a picture book) for themselves and even bring those objects to another ("Mommy, read to me.").

Reciprocally, standing and toddling infants seem more grown-up to adults, who, in turn, treat them differently. Thus, newly walking infants change their parents. Parents must now be vigilant about the possibilities that their baby may fall down steps, accidentally knock heavy things on themselves, or eat dangerous houseplants. Much more than before, parents must communicate to infants – primarily through their faces, voices, and gestures – messages that help infants regulate their own behavior and learn what to approach and what to avoid, not through potentially dangerous accidents but through the parents' emotional messages. For months, the baby was placed (helpless) in an infant seat or held in a caregiver's arms or straddled on a hip, with little need to curtail infant actions or reprimand the baby. Crawling and walking infants, by contrast, can get into trouble on their own ... and pretty quickly. Now, "No!" comes into the parent's vocabulary for the first time. Obviously, some infants crawl early, say by 6 months, whereas others may not until 9 months or even 1 year. In consequence, some babies are hearing socioemotional admonitions much earlier in their lives than others.

Indeed, many spheres of infant life are embedded in one another, like nested Russian dolls. For example, inner-biological factors are embedded in the individual infant, who is embedded in a family, which is embedded in a neighborhood, which is embedded in a community, which is embedded in a culture. At a given point in development, variables from any and all of these levels contribute to the status of structures and functions in infancy. In turn, these multiple levels do not function independently of one another; rather, they mutually influence one another (Kerig, 2019). To understand the contribution of different structures and functions to the whole of the infant as well as infant development, we treat growing, thinking, communicating, feeling, and relating in separate chapters in this book. However, along the way we set systems of growing, thinking, communicating, feeling, and relating in relation to each other, and in Chapter 7, we pull all these strands together into the fabric of a full systems perspective.

HOW INFANTS REVEAL THEIR SECRETS

For all of the reasons described to this point, people have long been fascinated by infancy and attended to infants. Infants are winning by their smiles alone, never mind that, if they do not survive, the human race ends. One can easily imagine the lengths to which cave parents went to keep their babies safe from all the threats and harms of living primitively in the wild. Paying attention to infants was the source of our first understandings of infants and in many ways ourselves. Parents, but also thinkers in philosophy and religion, have paid attention to babies and built grand theories of the nature of mind and morals on foundations of babyhood.

Infancy studies actually began with simple observations and diaries about babies (Box 1.4). However, for a science of infancy to progress, researchers needed to develop ways to overcome enormous practical and logistical challenges to studying infants – to get these nonverbal "little ones" (LO) to reveal their secrets. Perhaps the major challenge posed to developmental science was the fact that infants do not speak. Researchers trying to understand what infants might know and feel about the people and things around them must infer infants' capacities from small clues that infants' behaviors provide. As well, on account of their physical and psychological, emotional and verbal immaturity, **reliable** and **valid** measures of infant behavior have been challenging to craft. A reliable measure is one that can be used by multiple observers or across multiple assessments to obtain the same understanding (as a score or outcome). A valid measure is one that measures what we think it measures. Through the persistence and ingenuity of generations of developmental scientists, infants have given up many – but certainly not all – of their secrets. We discuss these methods in a bit of detail because what has been learned about infancy from developmental science springs directly from them. Understanding these methods leads to more deeply appreciating the substantive chapters in this book. Besides, we feel that the methods are also ingeniously fascinating in themselves.

So, how have babies been enticed to reveal their secrets? To begin to answer this question, a short digression is in order. There are two important principles of directionality related to infant physical and psychological development. First, development generally proceeds **cephalocaudally**, literally from head to tail, which means,

BOX 1.4   The Very Beginnings of Infancy Studies

The early philosophers and the first scientists based their conclusions about infants largely on observing infants and recording their observations. Rousseau was among the first to write about the integrity of early childhood as a separate stage of life. About the same time, the French lawyer and naturalist, Philippe Guéneau de Montbeillard (1720–1785) made a close analysis of the physical growth in his own son. Not long after that, the German philosopher Dietrich Tiedemann (1748–1803) wrote a psychological diary of the growth of a young child. His work became the first **baby biography**. Three types of baby biographies populate the literature (Wallace et al., 1994). Domestic diaries were typically written by mothers for their personal satisfaction and often provide insights into parental philosophies about the nature of childhood and childrearing. Educational diaries explore the impact of teaching or childrearing practices on children's behavior and development. Scientific diaries yield empirical knowledge about infancy and development. Both educational and scientific diaries came into their own when the British naturalist Charles Darwin (1809–1882), already famous as the author of *On the Origin of Species* (1859), published observations he had made in the early 1840s of his first-born son William Erasmus, nicknamed Doddy. Darwin's 1877 publication of *A Biographical Sketch of an Infant* simultaneously in German and English founded the study of infancy, and the attention paid to infancy by towering figures such as Darwin excited more general interest in children and in the study of children. Perhaps the greatest of the modern baby biographers was Piaget (1952, 1954), most of whose writing and theorizing about development in infancy refers to observations of his own three young children, Jacqueline, Lucienne, and Laurent. These first baby biographers documented basic information about development, and on the basis of their observations generated numerous novel and important hypotheses about infant development.

for example, that infants' heads, including their visual and auditory systems and their mouths, mature structurally and functionally before their upper extremities (arms), which, in turn, mature before their lower extremities (legs; Figure 1.4A). Second, development proceeds **proximodistally**, literally from close to far, that is from the center of the body to the extremities, which means, for example, that babies gain control over their necks before their arms and their arms before their fingers (Figure 1.4B). Taken together, these two principles pinpoint the brain, eyes, ears, and mouth as being the earliest structures to function in life.

To assess the capacities of infants, developmental scientists have taken full advantage of these twin developmental principles. To a great degree, the ingenious methods infancy researchers have relied

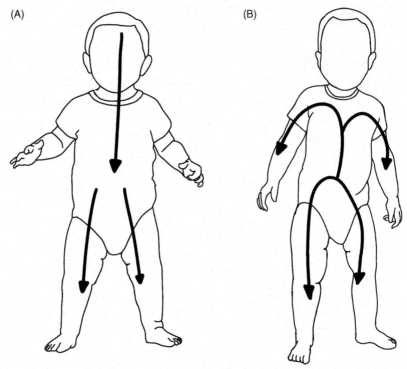

Figure 1.4 Cephalocaudal (A) and proximodistal (B) principles of development in fancy. (Created by A. E. Arterberry.)

on to discover what infants think and feel have called on measuring activity in infants' brains and calling on infants to look and listen. The various methodologies that researchers today use can also be organized into a taxonomy that reflects how much inference or assumptions different strategies demand in asking questions and seeking reliable and valid answers from infants.

DIARIES, INTERVIEWS, AND QUESTIONNAIRES

The earliest systematic information about infants did come from baby biographies (Box 1.4), but those diaries were often limited to just one child (generally case studies of the diarist's own baby) and usually the diarists themselves were writing about the child to make a point (e.g., like supporting their own philosophy). To find out about babies more scientifically and objectively, researchers developed variants of the biography method – issue-focused diaries, interviews, and questionnaires – in which parents provide information about their babies or themselves that will help answer specific research questions. For example, in a study designed to evaluate whether flexible work hours translate into more parental time with children, Baxter (2011) asked Australian working parents to keep weekday and weekend diaries describing the activities of their infants and with whom their infants interacted. The results showed that more flexible work hours allowed parents to distribute work and family activities, but it did not translate into more actual parental time with infants. Such diaries provide rich contextual information about infants' daily lives. More valid and reliable still are interview protocols and questionnaires. One type of protocol calls for parents to sort cards with statements on them into piles that describe attributes that are most characteristic or least characteristic of their infants (called a Q-sort; Belsky & Rovine, 1990). In this protocol, parents cannot just give socially desirable responses (answers they think the researcher wants to hear or that make them look good) because the piles must contain equal numbers of statements. This requirement enhances the reliability and validity of responses. Questionnaires are another widely used methodology. For example, the Infant Temperament Questionnaire asks parents about 191 (the long form) or 91 items (the short form) relating to their infant's temperament (Putnam et al., 2014), and the McArthur Communication Development Inventory asks parents to indicate the vocabulary words and word combinations their children know and know and produce (Fenson et al., 2000).

However informative, parental reports of these various types can be distorted. After all, what parent does not want their infant to look good? Moreover, diaries, interviews, and questionnaires as ways of studying babies are not actually measures of infants themselves. They are all measures of parents' perceptions of infants. Thus, diaries, interviews, and questionnaires are often used in combination with some type of objective descriptions by disinterested observers.

SYSTEMATIC OBSERVATIONS

Researchers use systematic observations of infants to gather information about infants' typical behaviors and daily lives. For example, naturalistic sampling is used to paint a picture of what infants normally do and what their everyday experiences are like. Investigators visit the home and observe and record (in real time or on video) anything and everything that go on in the infant's life. What feeding is like, how often it occurs, for how long, etc. Suppose, however, an investigator was interested in infant feeding, but during the time the investigator was in the home feeding never occurred. Because not all situations might arise during a naturalistic observation, an alternative strategy is to use standardized situations, in this case to ask the mother to feed her baby. Naturalistic sampling is especially revealing when studying infants in different cultures, and standardized situations are valuable when researchers want to understand how infants behave in different specific circumstances. Researchers who systematically observe infants naturalistically or in a systematic way use checklists, notebooks, or recorders in real time or electronic devices, video cameras, or computers to record behavior and analyze later. These two time-based procedures yield two sorts of measures: (1) simple indices of the frequency and duration of particular behaviors and (2) more nuanced indices of the likelihood that specific behaviors precede or follow one another. For example, Figure 1.5 shows that mothers engaged in mirroring most often to infant social behaviors and they matched negative affect with negative responses (such as "Oh, we cannot have that."). Many questions still can arise with observational methodologies, such as whether

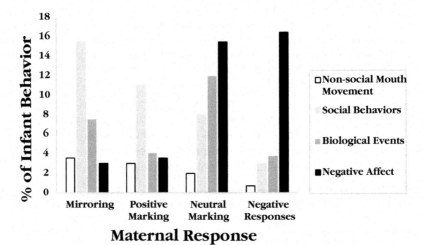

Figure 1.5 The percentage of time mothers responded to different infant behaviors within 2 seconds. Mirroring is making the same response as the infant, positive marking is smiling while singling out an infant response, neutral marking is singling out an infant response without smiling, and negative responses is criticizing, rejecting, or mocking the infant ("Oh, we cannot have that."). (From Murray et al., 2016; reproduced with permission.)

the behaviors observed are representative of the baby's general behavior (the window of the observation may not have been long enough or at the right time of the day to capture the relevant behavior) and whether the presence of the observer somehow distorted the infant's or mothers' behavior.

PHYSIOLOGICAL MEASURES

Diary, interview, questionnaire, and observational methods are revealing and provide rich but limited (and possibly distorted and sometimes only indirect) information. They also cannot tell us what the internal world of infants is like. Luckily, non invasive techniques allow researchers to gain access to the autonomic and central nervous systems of babies. The **autonomic nervous system** (ANS) is concerned with the structure and function of internal organs, including the heart, lungs, and digestive tract and also physiological responses. The brain and spinal cord comprise the **central nervous system** (CNS) concerned with processing information. Physiological measures from each system provide a window into physical, cognitive, verbal, emotional, and social development in infancy.

Activity of the autonomic nervous system includes heart rate and hormones. *Heart rate* is measured by attaching harmless electrodes (sensors with sticky tape) to infants' chests; it is an especially sensitive and revealing index of infant attention and emotion. For example, changes in heart rate indicate whether an infant is simply staring blankly at a stimulus (heart rate is stable) or attending to and processing information in the stimulus (heart rate slows noticeably during periods of concentration). Infants' heart rate reflects anger, excitement, or other affective displays as well. *Hormones* are chemicals released by a cell or a gland in one part of the body to send messages that affect cells in other parts of the body. Cortisol is secreted by the body at times of stress, and levels of cortisol (in saliva) are useful measures of acute (e.g., frightened by a jack-in-the-box toy) or chronic, ongoing stress (e.g., living in poverty).

Neuroimaging techniques provide a window onto the structure and function of the infant brain and sensory systems. One electrophysiological technique is the cortical *event-related potential* (ERP; Figure 1.6A). Electrodes placed on the scalp measure brain responses to stimulation, such as a face appearing on a TV screen. ERPs are fast and show the time course of information processing by the brain, the region of the brain where information processing is taking place, and the magnitude of the brain's response to information (when electrical

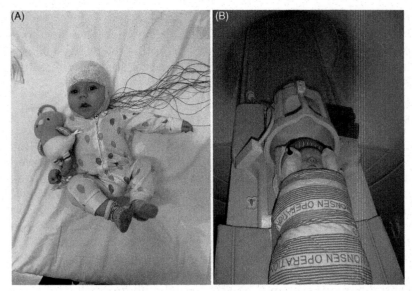

Figure 1.6 A. An infant wearing an EEG cap with sensors that record electrical activity at the scalp (Courtesy of M. H. Bornstein). B. An infant's brain activity is tested using fMRI, as reported in Fransson et al. (2007). (Courtesy of Karolinska University Hospital, Stockholm, Sweden.)

activity begins, where, and how much is going on). For example, in a study of memory infants were shown an object being hidden and ERPs recorded (Bell, 2012). Infants who remembered the location of the object showed a different pattern of brain electrical activity than infants who did not remember the object's location. ERPs as markers of brain maturation also predict later cognitive functioning.

Magnetoencephalography (MEG) is a second CNS technique to measure brain functioning. MEG has greater temporal and spatial sensitivity than EEG. For example, Ramirez and colleagues (2017) measured cortical MEG activity in 11-month-olds from both monolingual (English only) and bilingual (English and Spanish) families. Bilingual infants showed greater amounts of activation in more cortical areas than monolinguals, which may begin to account for cognitive advantages older child and adult bilinguals reportedly enjoy.

Functional magnetic resonance imaging (fMRI) and *functional near infra-red spectroscopy* (fNIRS) are two other CNS measurement techniques used with infants. Both identify regions of brain activity by scanning the brain and measuring subtle, ongoing changes in oxygen usage. (When the brain is active, regions involved in processing information use more oxygen.) These techniques provide accurate localization of specific brain activity. Because fMRI depends on putting the infant inside a tube surrounded by a strong magnet, and clear imaging is not possible when participants move their heads, fMRI has been used more with sleeping than awake infants (Figure 1.6B). For example, Blasi and colleagues (2011) presented sleeping 3- to 7-month-olds in an fMRI scanner with emotionally neutral, positive, and negative speech sounds as well as nonvocal environmental sounds. Infants' brains responded most to vocalizations, particularly sad ones, suggesting an early specialization for the human voice and negative emotions. fNIRS is more tolerant of movement, and infants may sit in a parent's lap during an fNIRS testing session. In one study, fNIRS revealed that 4-month-olds respond differently to male versus female voices, but only when the speakers used so-called child-directed speech, also known as "baby talk" (Sulpizio et al., 2018).

Physiological measures are thought to be objective and sensitive. They have also proved valuable in studying atypical development in infancy. For example, the ERP helps in the diagnosis of infant deafness: If the infant does not or cannot respond behaviorally to sound, the evoked potential at least helps to tell whether or not basic brain pathways are intact.

EXPERIMENTAL TESTING

As with many spheres of life, to know what infants know and what they can do requires further scientific investigation. Developmental scientists have created an impressive array of experimental techniques to assess the status and development of structures and functions in infancy. In doing so, they have taken full advantage of the twin principles of cephalocaudal and proximodistal development. Many experimental procedures used in infancy measure looking, listening, or sucking. Among these procedures, the most prominent kinds yield evidence of infants' natural preferences and different types of learning.

As anyone around babies knows, babies hardly hide their likes and dislikes. Babies' *natural preferences* are excellent tells about structure and function. Newborns given sweet, sour, or bitter substances to taste, and vanilla or raw fish to smell, all prior to the first time they have ever eaten, display different facial expressions to each (Figure 1.7). Within the first few months of life, infants show strong preferences for certain objects, simply by looking more at some than others. These kinds of preferences offer good evidence

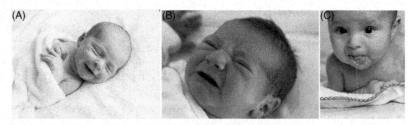

Figure 1.7 Infants' "gustofacial" responses to the taste of sweet (A), sour (B), and bitter (C). (Images courtesy of Shutterstock, copyright: Yulia Sribna/Shutterstock.com, Jorge Casais/Shuttertock.com and Dmytro Vietrov/Shutterstock.com.)

for function. If a baby is presented with two odors, raw fish to the left and vanilla to the right, and the baby regularly orients to vanilla, we can conclude that the baby can tell the difference between raw fish and vanilla smells, and prefers one over the other. Unfortunately, failure to demonstrate a preference does not indicate anything useful. An infant might look to mother and stranger equally, showing no preference, but still be able to tell them apart and may very well still prefer one to the other. Consequently, many investigators have turned to techniques that call on even more active infant behaviors. Among the most prominent are learning and habituation.

Like all living organisms, infants learn and therefore develop control over some of their behaviors. In **operant conditioning**, one type of learning, a naturally occurring behavior (sucking) is rewarded (with a sweet liquid) and as a consequence it tends to occur more frequently. Developmental scientists have used this kind of learning with a variety of infant behaviors, including sucking, eye movements, head rotations, and foot kicks, to gain access to infant perception and cognition. An example is a procedure that uses foot kicks and a crib mobile to investigate infant memory. The procedure unfolds in three phases (Figure 1.8). In Phase 1, infants lie in a crib with a mobile overhead. A ribbon is attached to the infants' ankle, but the ribbon is not connected to the mobile, so the infants' kicking does not cause the mobile to move (this phase serves as a baseline to measure rate of spontaneous kicking). In Phase 2, the learning phase, the ribbon is connected to the mobile so that the infants' kicks now cause the mobile to move, which is rewarding, and infants quickly learn the association between their kicks and mobile movement. Phase 3 is the test phase, and the ribbon is disconnected so again like Phase 1 the infants' leg kicks do not cause the mobile to move.

Baseline	Learning	Test

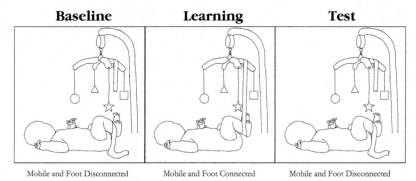

| Mobile and Foot Disconnected | Mobile and Foot Connected | Mobile and Foot Disconnected |

Figure 1.8 The setup for studying learning and memory using foot kicking. (Created by A. E. Arterberry.)

If infants remember that they could make the mobile move by kicking, then kicking during Phase 3 should be higher than the spontaneous baseline in Phase 1. Using this paradigm, researchers ask about infant memory, for example, such as how long can infants of different ages retain information. If the delay between Phase 2 and Phase 3 is a minute or an hour or a day, do infants remember (does kicking in Phase 3 exceed kicking in Phase 1)? Do infants remember if the context in which learning occurred (such as the colors and patterns on the crib bumpers) changes from the learning Phase 2 to the test Phase 3?

Just like adults, infants typically orient and look at a new stimulus, but if the stimulus remains visible or is presented repeatedly infants' attention diminishes. This reduced attention is called **habituation** (Figure 1.9) and suggests that infants recognize the repeated stimulus as the same as what they saw initially. Habituation is another type of learning. For example, it is reasonable to expect that older infants learn more quickly than younger infants, and so habituate more quickly; they do. Infants should also habituate to simple stimuli more quickly than to complex stimuli; they do. Interestingly, infants of the same age shown the same stimulus differ in habituating; that is, some habituate (learn) slowly whereas others habituate (learn) faster (we return to this individual difference later).

After habituation, infants can also be tested with the now familiar stimulus (the one from habituation) and a new (novel) stimulus (Figure 1.9). If infants remember the familiar stimulus, they should still find it boring and not look at it very long. If infants realize that they have not seen the novel stimulus before, they

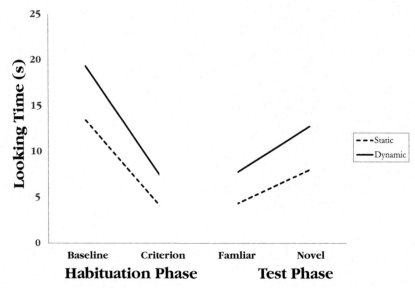

Figure 1.9 Looking to static and dynamic (moving) stimuli by 6-month-old infants. Baseline is the mean of the first two habituation trials, and criterion is the mean of the last two habituation trials (left side). Familiar is the same class of object as in the habituation (e.g., animal), and novel is a different class of object (e.g., vehicle). (Created by M. E. Arterberry with data from Arterberry & Bornstein, 2002.)

should look at it more than at the familiar stimulus. This recovery of looking to the new stimulus is known as **novelty responsiveness**, and it is quantified as the amount infants look at the novel stimulus relative to the amount they look at the familiar stimulus following habituation. In Figure 1.9, note that infants looked more to dynamic than static stimuli, but they became bored at the same rate in the habituation phase and they showed equal amounts of novelty responsiveness in the test phase. Developmental scientists have taken amazing advantage of this simple learning situation. For example, varying the difference between the familiar and novel stimuli tests how much change it takes for infants to notice two stimuli are different (such as the same face smiling or not to see if infants distinguish facial expressions of affect or two shades of blue to see if infants distinguish colors). The time between the end of habituation and the novelty test (again, a minute, an hour, a day) has been manipulated to evaluate how long memory for the familiar stimulus lasts.

TESTS

The final class of methods relies on babies' performance on actual tests. Most new parents will recall the very first test their baby took – twice, actually, once at 1 minute and once at 5 minutes after birth – the APGAR (which is an acronym for Appearance, Pulse, Grimace, Activity, and Respiration or the dimensions of newborn function the test assesses) and named after the developer U.S. physician Virginia Apgar (1909–1974). Generally speaking, tests include numbers of related items or simple tasks, and the infant is awarded a score based on the number of items or tasks completed successfully. The APGAR rates each of the five dimensions as 0, 1, or 2, and so 10 is a perfect score, but is rare at 1 minute after birth. For the Bayley Scales of Infant Development, another well-known infant test developed by U.S. psychologist Nancy Bayley (1899–1994), an infant's score for general development is the number of items successfully completed, and it is compared to the distribution of scores obtained from a nationally standardization group of infants of the same age.

In summary, developmental scientists have designed and implemented a variety of creative techniques from parent report to observation to neurological assessment to the application of experimental paradigms to overcome the major impediment infants present to researchers – their inability to speak. Even brief accounts of these procedures emphasize what they can and have revealed about infancy. However, each procedure has advantages and disadvantages, and these thumbnail descriptions have glossed over the shortcomings of each. For example, parent reports are based on those who have been with the infant the infant's entire life and know the infant best; but parents are not trained observers and (naturally!) want to see and tell you the best about their infant. Parent reports are also only indirect information about babies. Observations by trained observers can be direct and impartial, but there is no guarantee that an infant will display a particular behavior just at the time that the observer is present. That does not mean the infant is incapable of the behavior, however. Experiments are controlled, but experiments usually require specific equipment and laboratory settings, and many infants do not readily accommodate to the strictures of being experimental subjects. Tests are also objective and structured, giving each infant the same chance, but some infants are shy around strangers and do not perform as well as they could.

In consequence, the field of developmental science has come to value research that includes multiple assessments and converging research strategies in the use of reports, observations, experiments, and tests to be sure to overcome the shortcomings of any one procedure. Multiple assessments represent individuals better than single, brief assessments, and converging operations of two or more strategies permit investigators to select or eliminate alternative hypotheses as explanations for any single result.

Developmental scientists have also learned other important limitations to their work. Many limitations apply to infant assessment in the laboratory, but many also apply to everyday situations and parents need to be aware of them. Three examples that concern context, state, and the distinction between performance and competence illustrate the warning. First, laboratory research is not research in the home, and context matters. Infants might or might not behave the same way in different contexts, and so their behavior (ability, temperament, language) in one context should not be taken for their behavior (ability, temperament, language) generally. Babies might not be as chatty in the presence of researchers in the laboratory as they are in the bath with parents.

Second, one of the most important and ever-present influences on infant performance is behavioral state of arousal. Newborns and infants can (and do) shift rapidly and unpredictably from one state to another and may remain in a state of attentive alertness only for brief periods of time. Even when infant capacities are present and a task is well designed, infants' state may facilitate or interfere with performance. A baby who is awake, content, and attentive will have a better chance to perform well or participate more sensitively than one who is drowsy, hungry, and inattentive.

Third, there is a big difference between performance and competence. Performance concerns what infants *do* under certain conditions in certain contexts. However, such information does not tell us what infants *can do* in optimal circumstances; competence defines the infant's potential. Competence is often easily inferred from performance, but it is not necessarily the case that performance accurately indexes competence. Competence might far exceed performance. For example, babies understand a lot more language than they say. If we took babies' speaking vocabulary as an index of their knowledge of language, we would sorely underestimate them.

Nonetheless, in developing all these procedures and applying them to large numbers of babies in homes and laboratories around the world, an active generation of developmental scientists has unearthed important information about structures and functions in infancy and generated a substantial body of evidence-based literature about infancy and infant development. The secrets infants have divulged in these ways make up the contents of the chapters on growing, thinking, communicating, feeling, and relating that compose the rest of this book.

SUMMARY

Because of the range, the magnitude, and the implications of developmental changes that occur early in life, infancy is a fascinating and appealing phase of the life cycle. Some of the key issues in developmental science – those having to do with the relative importance of nature and nurture or with interrelations among diverse domains of development – are rendered in sharpest relief when the focus falls on infancy. Many theorists have asserted – and just as many have questioned – the status of infancy as a separate stage in the life cycle as well as the possibility of substages of development in infancy itself. Babies are particularly challenging research participants. They are mute, motorically inept, and subject to state fluctuations. Yet they are also important and attractive to study for a host of reasons. Most infancy studies are concerned with structures and functions as well as with their origins and developmental trajectories. This chapter introduced some background and some *hows* of infancy research; succeeding chapters turn to the *whats* and *whys* of infant development.

2

GROWING

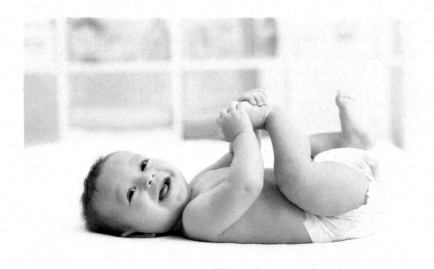

(Image courtesy of Shutterstock, copyright: Oksana Kuzmina/Shutterstock. com.)

INTRODUCTION

Infancy is a time of rapid growth. We practically see the infant emerging from the newborn and the toddler emerging from the infant before our very eyes. Each day brings dramatic changes. He

DOI: 10.4324/9781003172802-2

doesn't reach, and then he does. She doesn't turn over, and then she does. She doesn't follow my pointing finger, and then she does. One day he only grunts and gurgles, but the next he's making intelligible sounds. All of these advances come because of the interplay between physical maturation, particularly of the nervous system, muscles, and anatomical growth, and experiences.

Developmental scientists find it important to know about nervous system, physical, and motor development in infancy for at least two reasons. First, principles of development in these systems provide models for other domains of psychological development. The distinction between innate and congenital is an example. The term **innate** applies to structures and functions that are inherited, but may or may not be fully mature at birth. By contrast, **congenital** applies to structures and functions that are present at birth but are not inherited. Many characteristics are innate but not congenital because they emerge years later, at puberty for instance. By analogy, some mental abilities and emotional proclivities are innate but not congenital. Down syndrome is a congenital condition because it arises from too many chromosomes (as we explain later), but it is not inherited. Second, in the whole-child view, development of the nervous system, anatomy, and motor function influences the emergence and growth of other systems. Infants at first grasp small objects using the palm and whole hand, but only later pinch objects using the thumb and forefinger together. This gross-to-fine motor transition marks an advance in infants' tactile and visual inspection of objects, which, in turn, enhances exploration, learning, and cognition generally.

This chapter looks at topics of genetics, nervous system function, and physical development in infancy as important issues in themselves and explores how they pave infants' paths to development in thinking, communicating, feeling, and relating. Insights from genetics, anatomy, and birth deepen our understanding of infants' earliest capacities.

GENETICS AND DEVELOPMENT BEFORE BIRTH

Infant development begins long before birth. It was once believed that the infant is "preformed" in the mother's egg or in the father's sperm and just grew in size from there. We know now from modern biology that each parent's reproductive cells (**gametes**) contribute one member of each of the 23 pairs of **chromosomes** that compose the genetic makeup of their infant and that those chromosomes contain **genes** that are themselves composed of chemical codes of DNA that will guide development. Through fusion of the ovum and sperm, a full complement of chromosomes in the individual is again present.

Genes contribute critically – sometimes directly – to some aspects of life. For example, identifiable birth disorders, like hemophilia, are passed genetically from mothers to sons. Missing a chromosome or having an extra chromosome, as occurs in **Down syndrome** (or **Trisomy-21**, see Figure 2.1), is a genetic disorder. However, the **genotype** (the genetic makeup of the individual) does not always or even usually predict the **phenotype** (the observed characteristics of the individual). Direct and singular genetic determinism is very far from the rule. As we noted in Chapter 1, MZ twins with exactly the same genetic endowment might look or act very differently, just as organisms with different genetic endowments can look alike or act similarly (Figure 1.1). The individuality we see even in infants arises from many sources because genetics and experience together transact to shape the expression of all characteristics and behaviors of individuals. In keeping with a transactional perspective on development, not all growth before birth is genetically programmed. Many formative experiences arise from outside the womb; other experiences are produced by the developing fetus itself. Both types of experiences fundamentally influence pre- and postnatal development.

Physical growth before birth is standardly described as taking place in three main stages. The period of the **zygote** (the initial union of ovum and sperm) lasts from the moment of conception to 2 weeks, the period of the **embryo** from 2 weeks to 8 weeks, and the period of the **fetus** from 8 weeks to 40 weeks. (Oddly, pregnancy from the mother's perspective is more commonly divided into three equally spaced **trimesters** that do not map onto these scientifically defined periods of prenatal development.) These three periods mark important achievements and transitions in life before birth. Even by the end of the very brief zygotic period, human cells have begun to assume specialized roles depending on their location. During the embryonic period, organs, limbs, and other physiological systems like the skin, sense organs, and brain and spinal cord, muscles, blood, and the circulatory system differentiate (develop differently from each other). Embryos are proportioned according to the cephalocaudal principle (Figure 1.4): The head constitutes a much larger portion of total body size – between one-third and one-half of the entire length of the embryo – than it will at any other time in life. By the period of the fetus, differentiation of major

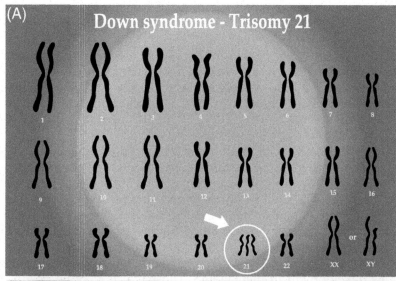

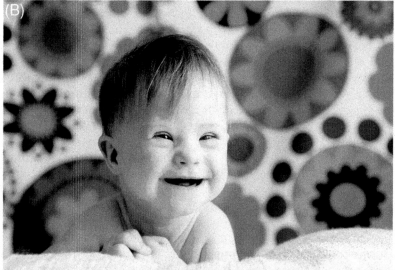

Figure 2.1 (A) The chromosomal makeup of a child with Down syndrome. Down syndrome is also known as Trisomy-21 because three, rather than two, chromosomes appear in position 21. (B) Down syndrome is associated with a variety of identifiable physical characteristics, including distinctive facial features, and with cognitive delay. (Images courtesy of Shutterstock, copyright: kanyanat wongsa/Shutterstock.com and Eleonora_os/Shutterstock.com.)

organs is complete, and the foci of development turn increasingly to structural growth and connections and to functions. During the fetal period, arms lengthen, joints develop, fingers separate, and a complex network of veins forms to nourish the cells while muscle connections lay the groundwork for finely coordinated limb movements. After 3 months, fetuses begin to swallow and urinate, by 4 months fetuses are felt to move *in utero* (**quickening**), by 6 months fetuses can breathe and cry, and by 7 months fetuses may survive (on their own) outside the womb.

It is a bit unsavory to think this way – but nonetheless a fact of life – that mothers-to-be are "hosts" to developing "organisms" – for example, measures of the maternal brain show clear shrinkage during pregnancy from before pregnancy and recovery of size after pregnancy attributed to the fetal organism "scavenging" nutrients from its host. This symbiotic relationship means that what mothers do – who they are, what foods they eat and drugs they consume, and what emotions and stresses they feel – influence that organism's development in their womb. Those effects may be positive or negative. Women who engage in healthy eating habits experience fewer complications during pregnancy, have shorter labors, and bear healthier babies. Mothers' activity is also a factor in prenatal development. Moderate walking, swimming, running, aerobic dancing, and riding a stationary bicycle for 30 minutes three times a week are recommended exercises for keeping mothers fit and supporting the developing infant's cardiovascular functioning. A study that monitored fetal heart rate of mothers who exercised found that, when mothers were at rest, their fetuses had lower heart rates and greater heart rate variability – both good things (May et al., 2010).

However, too large a proportion of the world's new mothers suffer malnutrition during pregnancy, and deficiencies in protein, zinc, and folic acid have been linked to certain birth defects. At the other end of the spectrum, mothers' weight gain is correlated with fetal weight, and too much weight gain during pregnancy is related to increased fat cells in children which may put them at risk for weight-related diseases like obesity later in life. Even parent age affects infant life before and after birth. Younger and older age in women increase the risk that their child will experience complications at birth. A study of over 8,000,000 live births to women aged 30–54 found that women who were 35 years of age or older were at higher risk for early birth (less than 32 weeks), prolonged labor, excessive bleeding, diabetes, and pregnancy hypertension than younger women (Luke & Brown, 2007). All things considered, as physicians have written at least since the 1740s, the ideal age for giving birth falls between a woman's 20s and 30s.

During intrauterine life, the fetus is protected from many (but not all) insults because the **placenta**, which connects host and organism via the umbilical cord permitting the vital exchange of nutrients and waste, also allows some harmful factors (**teratogens**) to reach the developing child. State, diseases, drugs, and environmental toxins pose particular threats to fetal integrity. Chronic stress during pregnancy is associated with premature labor and birthing complications. Various diseases – some all too common today like sexually transmitted diseases and HIV/AIDS – can also cross the placental barrier and affect the course and outcome of prenatal development (Box 2.1). As soon ago as 2018, it was estimated that worldwide over 1,000,000 children under the age of 9 were HIV positive, and the vast majority of them acquired the disease from an infected mother during pregnancy, labor, and delivery or through breastfeeding. The mother-to-infant transmission rate of HIV is about 15–45%. Fewer children today become infected with HIV because widespread public health efforts and the administration of anti-retroviral drugs have reversed this tragic situation.

BOX 2.1   Prenatal Exposure to Viruses

In November 2015, the Brazilian Ministry of Health declared a national health emergency due to an increase in infants born with microcephaly. Microcephaly is a condition characterized by a smaller-than-normal brain that is detected by measuring newborn head circumference (see Figure 2.2). The emergency was linked to the Zika virus (ZIKV), which is transmitted to humans by mosquitoes. According to Musso and colleagues (2019), the virus was first identified in Africa in 1947, and its first known appearance in the Americas occurred in 2015. In adults, exposure to the virus results in mild symptoms that last from 3 to 14 days, and people can spread the virus even when asymptomatic. The virus is transmitted during sexual contact from men to women, and the virus also crosses the placenta to embryos and fetuses where its effects are the most damaging during the first trimester. Nearly half of infants exposed to ZIKV *in utero* have abnormalities (Wheeler, 2018), but the most common, and most obvious, outcome is microcephaly. Due to the atypical development of the brain, these infants experience significant neurological insult, including severe motor impairment, seizure disorders, hearing and vision abnormalities, and sleep difficulties. Satterfield-Nash and colleagues (2017) found that ZIKV-infected infants fell far behind developmental age norms and predicted that these children would need ongoing support for the rest of their lives.

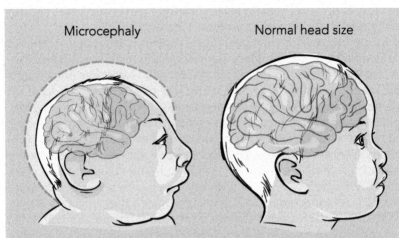

Figure 2.2 Head size and shape of a baby born with microcephaly compared to a normal baby. (Image courtesy of Shutterstock, copyright: Drp8/Shutterstock.com.)

The ZIKV health crisis calls to mind the novel coronavirus outbreak that began in late 2019 in China, resulting in world-wide infections of COVID-19. COVID-19 crosses the placenta, and exposure results in increased pre-term birth and pneumonia in newborns (Hamzelou, 2020; Yang et al., 2020; Zeng et al., 2020). The full picture of COVID-19's impact on infant development will not be understood for years after the pandemic when researchers can study the effects of exposure as a function of timing in the pregnancy and potential long-term outcomes. However, exposure to COVID-19 during pregnancy significantly elevates the risk for preterm birth, which in itself can have long-term consequences for infants (see Box 2.3).

Even the most well-meaning parents may not be able to protect their child from prenatal exposure to viruses. Close to 60% of adults in north eastern Brazil were infected with ZIKV (Musso et al., 2019). No one was prepared for the dramatic prenatal effects of this virus on the developing brain, on families, and on society.

Many pregnant women smoke tobacco, drink alcohol, or use illicit drugs. Nicotine from cigarette smoking constricts placental blood vessels, temporarily depriving the developing fetal brain of oxygen. Women who smoke have higher incidence of low birth weight and intrauterine growth retardation, and they place their children at risk for poor cognitive functioning. Excessive maternal alcohol consumption results in **fetal alcohol spectrum disorder** (FASD) involving physical malformation, growth deficiency, and central nervous system (CNS) dysfunction as well as impairments of cognition, social interaction, communication, personal living skills, and adaptive behavior in offspring. FASD is the leading cause of developmental delays with a known origin. Other illicit drugs, such as cocaine, heroin, and opioids, affect prenatal development and postnatal functioning detrimentally as well. Maternal prenatal cocaine abuse is associated with low birth weight, reduced head circumference and body length, high levels of irritability, poor state organization, and increased risk for **Sudden Infant Death Syndrome** (SIDS; that is, unexpected death within the first year of life). Longer-term effects of cocaine exposure are known to include intellectual and language deficits: Up to 40% of children whose mothers used cocaine pre- and postnatally have IQ scores of 85 or lower, well below the population mean of 100.

Prenatal exposure to drugs has both short- and long-term consequences for developing infants. In response, medical practitioners today are especially cautious about prescribing medications to pregnant women, and pregnant women are advised to consult with physicians before taking any medications, even those available "over the counter". In many countries, alcohol and tobacco packaging feature explicit warnings about the risks to pregnant women and their babies.

The teratogens just mentioned are avoidable, and exposure to them is by choice. Unfortunately, some teratogens are unavoidable and still pose toxic hazards for fetuses. PCBs (polychlorinated biphenyls), pesticides, mercury, and lead found commonly in the environment each has adverse implications for fetal and child development. PCBs once used widely in the electrical equipment industry are still present in the soil, water, and air and can be ingested by eating fish from contaminated lakes. Moreover, they can be transmitted from mother to baby via breastmilk. Prenatal PCB exposure is linked to lower birth weight, smaller head circumference, shorter gestation, poorer autonomic and reflex functioning, and long-term deficits in memory and language. We hope it is clear that teratogens are altogether insidious. Unfortunately, it is hard to eliminate all of them from one's life while pregnant. It is also hard to tell which of a number of possible sources of harm actually cause harm; we elaborate on this point in Box 2.2.

Fetuses also affect their own development. It is not possible to empirically "manipulate" human embryos and fetuses, but experimental studies with other species, such as chicks, demonstrate, for example, that immobilizing embryos results in muscle and joint abnormalities. Likely, chicks' own normal movements in the egg

BOX 2.2   Why Identifying the Effects of Teratogens Is Not Easy

Studying the teratogenic effects of diet, drugs, and other environmental toxins on the developing zygote, embryo, or fetus is complicated by several factors.

1. **The Dose-Effect Relations.** Sometimes, the mechanism of action of a teratogen is "linear" such that greater amounts (in dosages or exposures) are associated with greater effects in a regular relation. However, sometimes effects follow a "threshold" growth curve where outcomes only emerge when some fixed dose level is exceeded.

2. **Sensitive Periods.** Some teratogens have a damaging impact only at certain times in development but not at others. For example, alcohol consumption is more dangerous to the developing child in the first trimester of pregnancy than the last trimester.

3. **Sleeper Effects.** Some teratogens have immediate effects on development (such as cocaine and heroin on neonatal functioning), whereas others only show up later in childhood, such as a learning deficit or behavioral problem.

4. **Comorbidity.** It is difficult to pin down the effects of a single teratogen because one, such as alcohol use, may occur simultaneously with another, such as smoking, poor diet, and substandard housing with lead exposure. Which is responsible? Animal studies, in which there is a high level of control and fewer ethical concerns, can isolate the impact of a single toxin, such as the way nicotine induces DNA damage in mice. But in studies with human infants, researchers must rely on natural experiments or statistical techniques to try to isolate the effects of one teratogen from another. Moreover, it is likely that a child exposed prenatally to a nonoptimal environment will continue to experience a nonoptimal environment after birth. Consequently, it is difficult to determine whether a teratogenic effect is a product of one or another or a combination or continuing exposure to comorbid factors.

before hatching foster connections among developing cells. Human fetuses are very active, moving every 1–4 minutes as early as the second trimester, and fetal activity is related to the child's ability to regulate state of arousal after birth.

BIRTH

After approximately 280 days of gestation, some (still unknown!) factor causes the mother's pituitary gland to release a hormone (**oxytocin**) that, in turn, instigates expulsion of the fetus from her uterus. As the uterus is a muscle that expanded during pregnancy to accommodate the growing organism, **labor** involves involuntary uterine muscle contractions that literally force the fetus out. Contractions last 16–17 hours on average for first-time births. The narrowness of the vaginal birth canal leaves newborns looking red and battered with misshapen heads. (Babies normally arrive head-first, but sometimes they present feet or buttocks first.) Not all babies are born vaginally, for a number of reasons including health of the mother, health of the fetus, and fetal position. Alternative deliveries are by **Cesarean section**, a surgical procedure that involves cutting into the uterus to remove the baby. Among 4 million new births each year in the United States, full-term newborns measure on average 20 inches (51 cm) and weigh 6–9 pounds (2,700–4,100 grams). Most births are term (40 weeks), but others are early term (37–38 weeks), early and pre-term (less than 37 weeks), or late and post-term (over 41 weeks or later; Figure 2.3; Box 2.3).

Birth is a risky situation for mother and baby alike. In history, childbirth was a leading cause of death in young women (as headstones in any old cemetery attest). For their part, fetuses are at certain risk of oxygen deprivation (**anoxia**) because the umbilical cord can be pinched during a contraction or wrap around the baby's neck. A baby who is deprived of oxygen for more than a very short amount of time may suffer brain damage because brain cells require

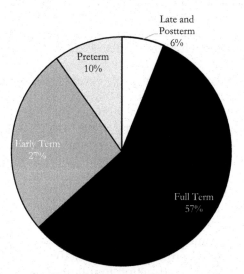

Figure 2.3 Births in the United States in 2018 as a function of gestational age. (Recreated from data provided by the Center for Disease Control and Prevention, https://www.cdc.gov/nchs/products/databriefs/db346.htm.)

BOX 2.3   Preterm Birth

Term infants are delivered about 40 weeks after the mother's last menstrual period. However, approximately 12% of babies are born early (Figure 2.3). An infant is preterm if born before 37 weeks gestational age, and of low birth weight if born under 5½ lb (about 2,500 g). Babies may be born preterm for a number of reasons, including abnormalities in the mother's reproductive system, poor health (including drug use, poverty, malnutrition, inadequate medical care, and unhealthy lifestyles), and age (teen mothers and mothers over the age of 35). Many multiple births (twins, triplets) are preterm. Babies who are preterm might be hospitalized for observation or to gain weight. Medical complications associated with prematurity include low birth weight and **respiratory distress syndrome** on account of preterms' underdeveloped lungs. To assist breathing, these "premies" are placed in incubators with high concentrations of oxygen. Preterm birth is also associated with **intraventricular hemorrhage** (bleeding in the underdeveloped brain) that risks later developmental and learning disabilities.

continuous oxygenation to survive and function. Brain cells are not usually replaced when they die, so damage to or loss of brain cells is often permanent.

From the baby's vantage, birth is both a process and an event. In one sense, birth continues development that unfolds along a maturing schedule, and CNS and motor structure and function are not really altered much by birth per se. Physiological characteristics like the infant's unique blood chemistry continue to emerge slowly over the entire course of gestation. As was the fetus, the newborn is dependent on others to maintain body temperature, for nourishment, etc. Yet, birth is a monumental event. With incredible suddenness, and for the first time, the organism separated from the host is responsible for its own circulation and respiration. Moreover, postnatal experiences impinging from all directions on vision, audition, smell, taste, and touch are new or radically changed from prenatal life.

Birth is also a monumental event for parents, as hormones, the brain, and behavior all change dramatically (and in many respects overnight) in both mothers and fathers. Hormones, like oxytocin in mothers and testosterone in fathers, activate key brain regions to increase new parents' attraction to infants' cues, induce positive mood, and render parents attentive and sensitive to babies' needs. Just 3 months of exposure to their own infant's face forges specific brain responses in new mothers (Bornstein et al., 2013). Similarly, their own infant's cries (compared to standard cries or control noises) result in specialized brain responses in new mothers and fathers (Bornstein, 2019).

Minutes after birth, the health and state of newborns in most U.S. hospitals are monitored with their first tests, administered right in the delivery room. The APGAR, mentioned in Chapter 1, documents normal functioning or determines any need for intervention.

Human newborns appear helpless, but evolution has prepared babies for extrauterine life with a small number of advantageous capacities. Some are simple, unlearned "stimulus-response" sequences (**reflexes**) that have survival value or adaptive significance (Figure 2.4). One kind of reflex is concerned with approach actions and includes breathing, rooting, sucking, and swallowing that maintain life. Another kind of reflex is concerned with avoidance actions and includes coughing, sneezing, and blinking to keep foreign substances or noxious stimulation away. Yet a third kind of reflex does not have obvious functions today, like the palmar grasp (the infant's tendency close fingers around something that touches the palm) and the Moro reflex (the infant's tendency to swing arms wide and then bring them together at the midline as if around the

Prenatal and Postnatal Reflexes

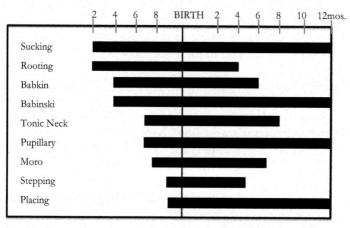

Figure 2.4 The variable appearance and disappearance of prenatal and postnatal reflexes. Some reflexes, such as sucking and rooting, appear very early in prenatal development, whereas others, such as stepping and placing, appear much later. Some reflexes, such as rooting and stepping, disappear early in postnatal development, whereas others, such as sucking and placing, persist well past the first year of life. (Created by M. E. Arterberry.)

body of a caregiver). These reflexes give the impression that they were important at an earlier point in human evolutionary history, and interestingly they still help many primate newborns keep close to their mothers by clinging to her body hair. Today, regularities in infants' reflexes provide a window on normal nervous system structure and function (just as general practitioner physicians test reflexes in adults during annual check-ups). On the one hand, reflexes have their origins in the deepest and most primitive parts of the nervous system, so their presence indicates normal neurological development, and their absence suggests neurological abnormality. On the other hand, most infant reflexes vanish in the second half of the first year as newer and more sophisticated brain processes come into play, so their eventual disappearance indicates normal neurological development.

PRINCIPLES OF PHYSICAL AND MOTOR DEVELOPMENT IN INFANCY

Physical growth in infants is readily observable and was a very early topic of study among the first baby diarists. Figure 2.5 shows Count de Montbeillard's 1759–1777 graph of his son's growth (still fairly accurate of children's development 250 years later!). Figure 2.5A tracks the boy's height year-by-year; Figure 2.5B plots the boy's growth in height each year. These graphs show two interesting growth spurts: one in the first year of life when the boy grew as much as 8½ inches (22 cm) in the year and a second around 14 years at the start of puberty.

The story of infant physical growth is significant for several reasons. The first is that growth data provide vital normative guidelines for healthy infant development. Every pediatrician's office has a growth chart for girls and boys hanging on the wall. A second reason is that, in the whole-child systems view of development, physical growth changes the direction of children's perceptual, mental, verbal, and social development (more about that later in this chapter). A third reason is that principles of physical development inform characteristics of the child's development in other psychological domains. Physical growth in infants actually illustrates at least five important principles of general development.

1. **Directionality.** As we introduced in Chapter 1, growth of anatomy (structure) and complexity of voluntary control (function) both follow cephalocaudal and proximodistal directions in development (Figure 1.4). A third direction is

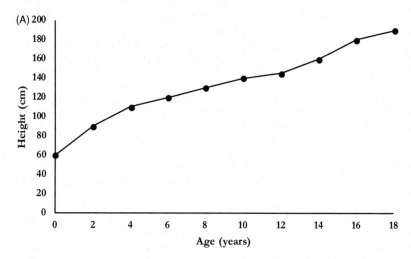

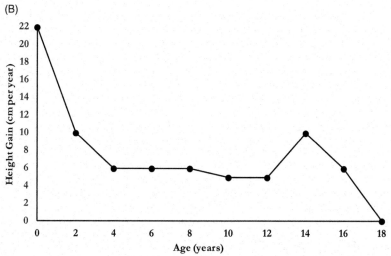

Figure 2.5 The growth of the son of Count Philippe de Montbeillard from birth to the age of 18 years. (A) Height he reached at each age and (B) annual increments in height. (From Tanner, 1962; reproduced with permission.)

mass-to-specific, that is from larger muscle groups to finer ones: Infants move their arms before they are able to make a pincer thumb movement or wiggle a forefinger.

2.   **Independence of Systems.** Different domains of development are in different states of maturity in infancy and develop along different trajectories through the first 2 years of life

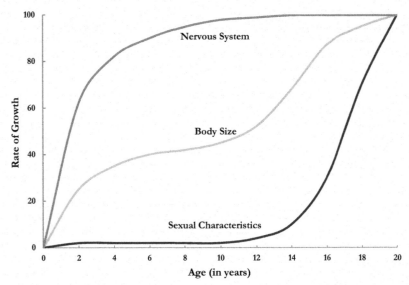

Figure 2.6 Growth of different bodily systems as a percentage of adult status. In infancy, the nervous system is highly developed, body size is less developed, and secondary sexual characteristics are least developed of all. (Created by M. E. Arterberry.)

(Figure 2.6). By 2 years, for example, the nervous system has achieved more than one-half of its adult status, whereas physical characteristics of the body have developed to less than one-third of their eventual mature state, and, of course, secondary sexual characteristics have hardly developed at all.

3. **Canalization**. Certain systems seem to be protected in the sense that their developmental outcome is assured even under less than optimal initial circumstances. So, preterm infants born diminutive in length and low in birthweight eventually catch up in physical development to children their age in the general population.

4. **Norms**. The average height of a U.S. European American male is 5 feet 9 inches (175 cm). Most adults are 5 feet to 6 feet tall, and very few are either 4 feet or 7 feet tall. Height is distributed in the population in a statistically *normal* fashion, that is according to the well-known bell-shaped curve with a peak at the average and tapering toward the two extremes. Like height, many biological and psychological characteristics are normally distributed. The average is often taken to represent the distribution, but the range and form of the distribution

are critically informative about every structure and function. This point cannot be stressed enough with regard to infancy. Every parent looks for signs of development in their baby: Reaching, turning over, following a pointed finger, responding to their name, and on and on. In doing so, parents use the average age at which these milestones are achieved. However, individual babies do not know the average, and the average may actually apply to only a small proportion of babies. The age at which infants first walk or talk has enormous psychological importance, but the true range is extraordinary, especially when considered as a proportion of the child's age. Some children first walk at 10 months, others at 18 months; some children say their first word at 9 months, others at 29 months. In the end, timing may be meaningful only for very extreme cases. All adults can generally walk and talk, so the exact onset of an infant's walking or talking might be less meaningful in the long run than vigilant (or worried) parents often think. Norms are the averages for a population, but they are descriptions rather than explanations; they represent likely outcomes rather than actual or even ideal outcomes.

5.   **Individual Differences**. Every infant is a unique combination of biology and experience, the continuing transaction of nature and nurture. Typically developing infants are likely to fall anywhere in the normal distribution. In addition, individual differences and their transactional causes mean that infants can follow any one of many different paths in development. Different infants might develop at different rates but eventually reach the same mature level; different infants might develop at the same rate but stop developing at different final levels; and different infants might develop at different rates and reach different final levels. These diverse developmental trajectories also can have many causes. Infants in resource-rich countries tend to be healthier, heavier, and longer than infants in resource-poor countries, presumably reflecting differences in genetic variation, prenatal and postnatal nutrition and care, and maternal health and education. By the end of the first year of postnatal life, the average infant in the United States weighs about 20 pounds (9 kg) and is about 30 inches long (76 cm). However, even within affluent countries such as the United States, children born into low socioeconomic status families have lower birth weight, but they are at a higher risk for obesity later in life.

TWO INFANT NERVOUS SYSTEMS

The human nervous system is particularly remarkable and infinitely complex: It is estimated that adult human brains house perhaps 100 billion cells (**neurons**). Surprisingly, however, relatively few neurons are believed to be created after birth. Dividing 100,000,000,000 by 9 months of gestation × 30 days per month × 24 hours per day × 60 minutes per hour = 388,800 minutes means that an average of more than 250,000 new brain cells are created every minute of prenatal life. In a short 270 days, a single fertilized egg evolves into the astonishing nervous system that supports the infant in thinking, communicating, feeling, and relating during the additional 18 months after birth ... and most all that the person will learn for the rest of life.

We need to lay a little groundwork before coming to describe how very important the two nervous systems are to infant development; after all, together they comprise all the neural tissues in the human body. From a structural point of view, the nervous system has central and peripheral components. The central nervous system (CNS) comprises the brain and spinal cord, and connections of receptors (such as the eye) and effectors (such as the muscles) to the brain. From a functional point of view, the nervous system has somatic and autonomic components. The **somatic nervous system** is concerned with voluntary control of body movements via skeletal muscles (which we discuss later in this chapter in the section on motor development), and the **autonomic nervous system** (ANS) is concerned with automatic and non voluntary processes.

THE INFANT AUTONOMIC NERVOUS SYSTEM

The fetus and the newborn are biological organisms. They are more about survival and less (if at all) about conscious or voluntary activity. Two principal considerations regarding ANS function in infancy are, first, cycles and states (such as wakefulness and sleep) and, second, development of the heart. Looking ahead, the issue of cycles and states anticipates the key development of self-regulation in infants. It turns out that the heart constitutes a window on the infant mind.

If you were to sit back and watch a newborn baby, say, over the course of a day, you might be very impressed by what appears to be a lot of spontaneous, disorganized, and sporadic activity. Babies constantly move their eyes, hands, and feet without any apparent purpose, and over longer periods they shift randomly and unpredictably between sleep and alertness. However, looks deceive the untrained eye. Close and consistent inspection (which is what developmental scientists do for a living) reveals that infants are subject to regular patterns or rhythms. Some rhythms are **endogenous** or naturally occurring and are thought to be driven by "pacemaker" cells in the brain; other rhythms are **entrained** or learned through the experiences infants have. For example, preterm newborns who receive extensive skin-to-skin contact show more quiet sleep than those who do not. Contingent and responsive caregiving anticipates better state regulation beginning as early as the first 10 days of life. Newborns receiving responsive care (according to infant cues) develop more regular patterns of sleeping, feeding, and elimination compared to newborns receiving regularly scheduled care (feeding, diaper changes, social interaction).

Why then do infants seem so chaotic in their activity? Endogenous activity in infants is actually organized at fast, medium, and slow cycles or rhythms. Some activities cycle at high frequencies (appear and disappear, increase and decrease) every second or so (Figure 2.7A). Heartbeats, breathing, and sucking exemplify fast rhythms that maintain life. Other general bodily movements cycle at intermediate or

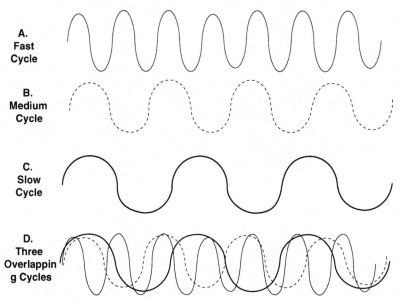

Figure 2.7 (A) Fast cycle. (B) Medium cycle. (C) Slow cycle. (D) Representation of the seeming chaos of overlapping fast, medium, and slow cycles. (Created by M. H. Bornstein.)

medium rates, on the order of once every minute or so (Figure 2.7B). Still others like states of arousal (sleep, drowsiness, alertness, distress, and activity) cycle at slow frequencies (Figure 2.7C). Piled on top of one another, fast, medium, and slow cycling states can give the impression of chaotic baby activity (Figure 2.7D).

In short, apparent randomness and unpredictability may be only just that, apparent. Sleep–wake patterns change over the course of the life cycle. Newborns typically wake when they are hungry, and not long after feeding they go back to sleep, resulting in their sleeping approximately 16 hours per day. Across the first year of life, infants spend less and less time sleeping such that by 1 year of age they sleep perhaps half the day with a nap during the day and one long sleep at night. Infants may take months to establish a predictable sleep–wake cycle.

On the whole-child view, the amounts of time and predictability of infant states have wide implications for infant development. Whether and how infants respond to tactile, visual, and auditory stimulation depends on their state. Infants who are awake and alert can engage in play and learning. In quiet alertness, an infant may attend to a voice that has no effect on the same baby when crying. Adults rock and soothe distressed babies instead of trying to show them toys. Infants who are predictable in their cycling allow their caregivers to adjust their own interactions optimally to the infant's development. In this transaction, infants affect their own development by affecting how and how often others respond to them. The regularity of infant state also serves as a marker of nervous system maturity and integrity. Poor state regulation is common among less well-developed infants (such as those born preterm), and poor state regulation in early infancy is a risk factor for SIDS.

The human heart begins to beat early in the period of the embryo. At first, heart rate is rather constant, suggesting that strong endogenous pacemakers are at work. After birth, heart rate is extremely sensitive to psychological state and (as noted in Chapter 1) has been used to help interpret what infants might be thinking or feeling. Notably, deceleration in heart rate indexes sustained visual attention and reactivity to psychologically meaningful stimulation. Heart rate can be assessed noninvasively from the **electrocardiogram** (ECG). One study measured heart rate when 13½-month-old infants interacted with a stranger with or without their parent present (Hill-Soderlund et al., 2008). Infants who showed no outward signs of distress when their parent left them alone with the stranger nevertheless showed changes in their heart rate that resembled changes that infants show when they are experiencing distress. From this study we learn two lessons. One is that infants might experience internal distress in the absence of their manifesting external distress. The other is that infants who show few outward behavioral signs of distress might rely on self-regulation to a greater degree than other infants of the same age who show more outward behavioral signs of distress. As we have seen, the ANS serves regulatory functions early in prenatal life and involves regular cycles and states of arousal after birth. Both cycles and states impact other psychological characteristics of developing infants and their parents.

THE INFANT CENTRAL NERVOUS SYSTEM

The CNS is largely concerned with processing environmental information and controlling voluntary activity. The CNS develops simultaneously at multiple levels – from miniscule cellular to larger brain structures. It is incorrect to think that development of the CNS follows a strictly maturational program. To be sure, the CNS is a biologically unfolding system, but its development is also exquisitely shaped by experience.

Again, a little foundation laying is in order. Figure 2.8 shows a single **neuron**, including the cell body, nucleus, dendrites, axon, myelin sheath, and synapse. The cell nucleus housed in the cell body contains DNA, the basic information of life. **Dendrites** carry information from one cell to another cell. (When cells are active

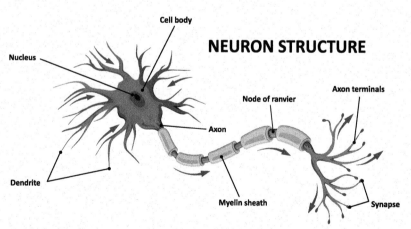

Figure 2.8 A single neuron showing the cell body and nucleus, dendritic fibers, and the axon, surrounded by a myelin sheath, and flow of the action potential, indicated by the arrows. (Image courtesy of Shutterstock, copyright: logika600/Shutterstock.com.)

it is called "firing.") **Axons** (which can be infinitesimally short or up to 3–4 feet [1 m] long) transmit information away from the cell body to other cells. Undeveloped cells are nude; developed cells are wrapped in a sheath of a fatty tissue (**myelin**) that speeds information conduction along the axon. That information eventually reaches axon terminals that conduct the information to other cells' dendrites across **synapses**. Information crosses synapses via chemical **neurotransmitters**.

The CNS originates as a cell layer on the outer surface of the embryo, and this layer is already visible 1 month after conception. After neurons are born, they grow, send their axons to other cells, and eventually associate with one another to create interconnecting patterns. Four aspects of cellular development are noteworthy, and each is startling. First, recall that the brain generates upwards of one-quarter million cells per minute prenatally. Second, in a still deep mystery of brain development, routes that axons follow to connect cells seem to be predetermined (cells "know" their partners and can "find" them). Moreover, the generation of synapses occurs at different times accounting for changes in function with age. Third, structural myelination loosely correlates with the development of function. With myelination the velocity of neurotransmission along a cell axon triples from less than 20 feet (6 m) per second to more than 60 feet (18 m) per second. Myelination does not occur all at once. Neurons concerned with vision and audition myelinate before birth, whereas neurons in higher brain centers are not completely myelinated until well into puberty.

Fourth, dendrites and axon terminals grow spines to connect cells, a process that resembles trees with branches and roots and is aptly called **arborization**. This vital feature of human brain growth is illustrated in Figure 2.9A. In just the first 2 years of life, arborization circuitry makes up to 10,000 connections per cell. At first, synapses are overproduced in many parts of the brain. Soon, however, synapses are eliminated in a process (following the forestry metaphor) called pruning, illustrated in Figure 2.9B. Many explanations for cellular overproduction and subsequent elimination have been suggested. Perhaps limited space in the skull forces the elimination of many connections. Perhaps neurons initially send out lots of connections, but not all neurons connect successfully to their appropriate targets. Perhaps neurons reduce the number of their connections to support more efficient information transmission in those that remain. Perhaps cellular activity itself establishes and maintains certain neural circuits, with different activities determining which synapses are retained and which eliminated.

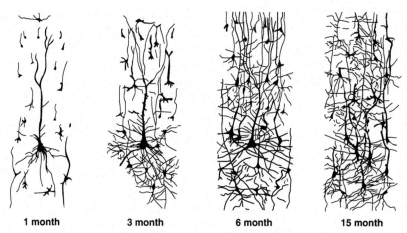

Figure 2.9A Illustration of dendritic arborization from 1 to 15 months of age. (Courtesy of J. L. Conel; redrawn for clarity.)

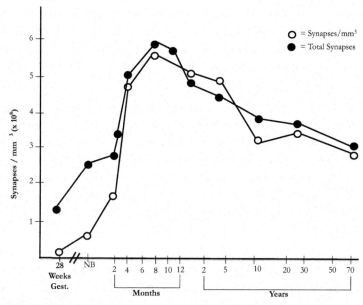

Figure 2.9B Synapse counts in layer 3 of the middle frontal gyrus of the human brain as a function of age. Note the rapid increase in synapses through the first year of life and the decrease by puberty and into old age. Reprinted from *Neuropsychologia*, *28*(6), Huttenlocher, 1990, Morphometric study of human cerebral cortex development, 517–527, with permission from Elsevier.

The last explanation for the overproduction-elimination cycle represents a famous principle of brain cell development, *cells that fire together wire together* (Hebb, 1949). Here is a simplistic but not altogether inaccurate way to think about brain development in this regard. When people think or act in a certain way, their brain is of course involved. The way it is involved is that connections are made between cells. If a thought pattern or action is repeated, the paths between cells involved in that thought or action connect. The more the thought or action is repeated, the stronger the path connection between them. Imagine two villages separated by some fields and hills. At first, villagers who want to travel from one to the other make their own way across the fields and hills. Soon, however, villagers discover the paths of least resistance (those that are shorter and easier to walk or navigate) and those paths become used more, whereas the paths that are more difficult (those over higher hills or across always marshy fields) become used less. Travel across some paths eventually disappears altogether, and the frequently used paths grow in efficiency and first become walkways, then streets, and then highways.

The result is that cells and connections in the brain that are used together to complete a thought or action are retained, and those that are not are eliminated. Thus, development in the CNS is fostered by positive active experiences. Regardless of the reason for overproduction and then pruning, in time the seemingly haphazard immature pattern of multiple intercellular connections is replaced by an efficient and streamlined information transmission system. By way of illustration, consider how younger versus older babies respond to a loud clap. Early in life, a sudden auditory stimulus like a clap elicits a gross response, like a whole-body shudder. Later, however, the same clap leads to a discrete and efficient turn of the head. Experiences promote the organization of assemblies of cells, and metabolic changes via neurotransmitters facilitate connections among cells to promote efficient pathways of information transmission. Relevant regions of the brain become more finely tuned and connected as a function of repeated experiences.

As cells in the brain aggregate and become organized, cell masses soon give the brain its characteristic wrinkly appearance of hills (9 **gyrus**), flatlands, and valleys (**sulcus**). Different structures of the brain control different functions. Evolutionarily older more primitive parts of the brain that control state and arousal emerge first in development: The **reticular formation** governs sleep/wake cycles, and the **limbic system** governs emotion and behaviors needed for survival, such as feeding. Evolutionarily newer parts of the brain develop later (some are not fully developed until a person's 20s):

The **cortex** and **cortical association areas** are concerned with awareness, attention, memory, and the rich processing of information. The cortex has four main lobes or regions of function (Figure 2.10). The **occipital lobe** processes visual information; the **temporal lobe** governs auditory processes and language; the **parietal lobe** registers temperature, taste, and touch and directs motor movements; finally, the **frontal lobe** is the center of higher-order cognition and controls voluntary activity. These cortical regions are also the last to myelinate, and they are influenced most by experience with the world outside the brain.

The brain has two **hemispheres** connected by a bundle of neurons called the **corpus callosum**. It is among the last CNS structures to develop and myelinate. Research with adults who have had their hemispheres surgically disconnected by cutting the corpus callosum (to stop the spread of electrical seizures across the brain as in epilepsy) indicates that the brain's two hemispheres roughly divide

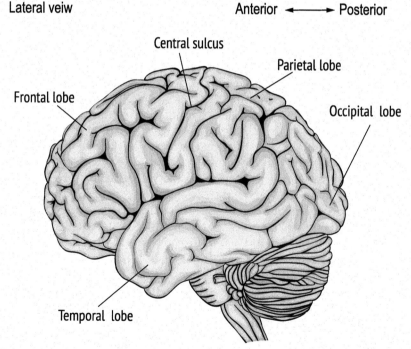

Figure 2.10 The human brain contains four cortical lobes on the left and right sides. In this image the eyes are to the left (the frontal lobe is at the front of the head). (Image courtesy of Shutterstock, copyright: Vasilisa Tsoy/Shutterstock.com.)

mental duties. Language is processed predominantly in the left hemisphere and spatial information in the right hemisphere. Also, normally the left half of the brain controls the right half of the body, and the right half of the brain controls the left half of the body. The consequences for infant development of these startling facts of brain geography must be profound, but developmental science has yet to explore and understand them fully.

It is, of course, not possible to observe or to measure brain activity directly human infants. However, developmental scientists have figured out ways to assess structural and functional growth indirectly using some of the methods and techniques we introduced in Chapter 1. EEG recordings that reflect spontaneous electrical activity over masses of individual cells under the scalp is one. Figure 1.6 shows EEG being assessed in a baby. In broad outline and to be expected, over the course of the first year of postnatal life brain activity becomes increasingly mature in terms of speed, regularity, and strength. Moreover, increases in activity over the different structures of the cortex (for example, the frontal area) parallel changes in function (such as the growth of cognition). Such results are informative, but far from offering determinative or key information about brain development in infancy. For example, they leave unanswered the direction of these effects. Do thinking and experience propel neurological development, or does maturation of neurological structures govern improvements in thinking?

ERPs are averages of EEG activity and allow us to characterize a specific pattern of brain activity evoked by a specific stimulus. ERPs also provide valuable information about development of the brain. For example, if we flash a picture of a face (for, say, 5 seconds), the adult ERP shows a quick response in the visual cortex (around 170 milliseconds after the start of the presentation); this ERP indicates a face has been perceived. Other stimuli, such as houses or plants, do not evoke this type of response. If the face is familiar, the ERP shows a distinctive profile around 300 milliseconds, and this profile is different from the one seen for unfamiliar faces. Infants early in life also show this pattern, although the response is not as strong (the amplitude is not as high) and it takes longer (latency). ERPs have also been used to determine whether and when babies sense sounds. At the onset of a sound, a baby may or may not orient to it behaviorally. However, an infant's nonresponse to a sound may not definitively indicate whether the baby has heard the sound. ERPs can show that the infant's brain responds to the sound. In one study, infants were played a simple "pa" sound on 80% of trials and a "ba" sound on the remaining 20%. Infants' ERPs showed different patterns to the more frequent "pa" and the less frequent "ba" indicating that the infants' brains discriminated the two sounds (Pivik et al., 2011).

EXPERIENCE AND THE INFANT BRAIN

As this description attests, CNS development is vital to life. (Religion once marked the end of life by the end of breathing; medical science today marks the end of life by the cessation of brain activity.) Moreover, the preceding discussion might suggest that CNS development in prenatal and early postnatal life is fairly regular and likely preprogramed. However, brain development is far from fixed. Experiments with animals (such as monkeys whose early structural brain development is faster but otherwise not so different from that of humans) and with human infants indicate that experience matters a lot to normal development and that specific experiences matter to specific aspects of development. Consider one example. All babies, regardless of whether they can hear or not, begin to babble around the middle of the first year of life. Typically developing hearing babies hear language around them and hear their own babbling, and they continue to babble. Moreover, their early sounds eventually emerge as words. In the absence of hearing experience, deaf babies stop babbling. Thus, for both hearing and deaf babies, the brain is prepared to foster language development, but without general exposure to language, development stalls.

Specific experiences with specific stimulation also matter. Specific experiences modify brain structure and influence brain function and, importantly, contribute to individuality. Enrichment and deprivation illustrate such specific-experience effects, and both affect the fine and gross structure of the nervous system as well as functional properties of cortical neurons. An example of enrichment in human infants is bilingualism. Children exposed to more than one language from birth enjoy different linguistic experiences from those exposed to only one language, and bilingually developing infants show different ERP profiles to verbal stimuli from monolingual children (Conboy & Mills, 2006). Thus, enriching exposure to more than one language early in life influences brain development.

An example of deprivation effects on neural development comes from studies of orphans (Box 1.2; Moulson, Fox, et al., 2009; Moulson, Westerlund, et al., 2009). In the Bucharest Early Intervention Project, three groups of children were compared for their neural responses to faces: children who had lived their whole lives in an orphanage (institutional care group), children who had experienced an orphanage but were placed in foster care between 5 and 31 months of age (previously institutionalized group), and children who never experienced institutional care (never-institutionalized group). Children in institutionalized care have fewer opportunities to engage with people and to see a variety of different faces. To assess children's neural responses to faces, all children in the three groups were shown images of familiar and unfamiliar faces and their brain responses were measured at several time points across the first 3½ years of life. Institutionalized children showed underdeveloped ERPs, and children who were placed in foster care showed increases in ERP development after placement (suggesting also that early effects of social deprivation can be reversed). In light of the different kinds of information and different sources of experience, it becomes clear that brain structure and function alike are plastic and moldable. CNS development is jeopardized by other adverse life experiences as well. Chronic maternal prenatal alcohol consumption inhibits fetal brain formation of axons and dendrites and cell migration. Lead exposure (as from paint) damages nerve cells and myelin. And exposure to ZIKV caused profound CNS damage (Box 2.1).

In general terms, infant brains come into the world ready to respond to and be shaped by critical experiences and features of the environment. Brains adapt to experiences and environments in which they find themselves. Moreover, windows of brain modifiability open in infancy so that the brain can prepare quickly and efficiently for the particular experiences and features of the environment in which it will develop and needs to succeed.

Clearly, the nervous system underpins the many remarkable accomplishments of infants. However, it is difficult to establish strict causal relations between brain and behavior, structure and function. There are several reasons for this. First, as alluded to earlier, brain–behavior relations are bidirectional. Genetically predetermined brain development may permit new behaviors that generate new interactions with the environment, but experience then feeds back to influence brain development. Consequently, neurological growth always reflects the dynamic interplay of genetic influences and selected (including self-generated) experiences. Second, much of developmental scientists' knowledge of early neurological development derives from studies of nonhuman organisms, and developmental scientists are cautious about applying that knowledge willy-nilly to human beings. All biological systems do not look the same in different species, develop the same in different species, or work the same in different species. Third, behavior normally has multiple causes. Certainly, the brain is intimately involved in motor function, but so is parenting, culture, and opportunity.

Brain–behavior interactions are complex, but it would be surprising if development was not reflected in parallel changes in brain structure and function.

In the story of CNS development, the vital role of experience is clear. Experiences arise from many quarters. Parents provide infants with most of their experiences. So do the material world, social class, and culture. Cultural experience is especially telling in infant development. Indeed, one anthropologist contended that *the* most significant factor in one's life is the culture (place or nation) where you are born and now live. Even birth itself reflects cultural context. Shostak (1981) wrote a biography of a !Kung woman living in the Kalahari Desert of Africa in the middle of the 20th century. At the time of delivery following the way of her people, the mother simply walked alone a short way out of the village, squat against a tree, and gave birth. As we write, the world is haunted by the image of a very pregnant Ukrainian mother being carried on a stretcher from the ruins of a maternity hospital bombed by Russians. As the story is told, when the mother learned in the very next days that her baby did not survive, she too tragically passed.

INFANT MOTOR DEVELOPMENT

Infants' abilities to coordinate physical movement develop impressively over the first 2½ years. Movements that seem uncontrolled for the first few months coordinate rapidly thereafter. Newborns are unable to roll over from wherever placed, but toddlers are increasingly deft, so much so that parents quickly learn that they must constantly monitor their 2-year-olds' activities and whereabouts. In motor development, as in other spheres of infant life, infant and environment work in tandem to optimize or retard development.

It will come as little surprise at this point that the sequence and coordination of motor development in infancy depend on both biology and experience. On the one hand, motor development reflects the sheer growth of strength and organization of limbs and muscles to act in a coordinated fashion. Two related neurological systems direct motor activity: The **pyramidal system** controls precise, rapid, and skilled movements of the extremities (such as walking), and the **extrapyramidal system** controls posture and coordination. These neuromuscular systems begin developing early in the second trimester of pregnancy. As they further develop after birth, the infant is increasingly able roll over, sit upright, crawl, and manipulate objects. In the normal course of things, all these accomplishments appear seamless and natural in their emergence. They arrive, however, under the watchful eyes of parents concerned with infants meeting regular motor milestones. Despite seeming regularities of motor development, it is not the case that infants automatically achieve more sophisticated and complicated motor feats as they simply mature physically. Rather, experiences deeply influence the course of motor development, and children's own movements, even as a fetus, feedback to enhance or inhibit their motor development. In this connection, the value of multidisciplinary developmental science is especially instructive. Another poster common in pediatricians' examination rooms, in addition to height and weight charts, displays motor milestones of the first years. Babies are expected to roll over at such and such an age, put a cube in a cup at such and such an age, and begin to "cruise" by toddling while holding on to a support at such and such an age. These milestones date back to the painstaking observations of Gesell, who (recall from Chapter 1) filmed and closely analyzed the motor development of local New Haven, Connecticut babies over the first years of life. On the basis of his extensive and careful observations, he then averaged infants' accomplishments and codified those well-known guidelines of what normal infant development at different ages entailed.

We called out a warning about the dangers attendant to placing too much credence on norms earlier in this chapter. Here is another. After WWII, infant testing reached beyond New Haven and the middle-class European American society that it served. The results of cross-cultural surveys among indigenous peoples in North America, in Southeast Asia, and in Africa revealed that babies in these different cultures deviated from those accepted "universal" Gesell milestones with respect to both the stages and the timing of motor development. Native American Hopi infants begin to walk alone later, African Ghanda and Wolof infants are more advanced in motor development, and Balinese infants follow different stages on their way to walking. In each case, infants' motor achievements reflected their specific experiences. Indeed, walking is a learned activity and can be taught. Experiments demonstrate that an early start and extra practice advance motor development in otherwise typically developing infants. Likewise, natural experiments in different cultures confirm that motor retardation in African Baoulé infants, relative to French children both growing up in Ivory Coast, Africa, is accounted for by the fact that African Baoulé babies are carried on their mothers' backs. In addition, African Kipsigis mothers deliberately teach their infants to sit, stand, and walk, which the infants do surprisingly early; but Ghanda and Kipsigis African infants reared in the manner

of European babies lose the motor advantages that their traditionally reared, genetically similar compatriots enjoy. These kinds of cultural differences are hardly quaintly antiquated: a 2019 study found
that the average age at which Dutch babies walk independently is
about 2 months behind their Canadian peers (Suir et al., 2019). Infant
motor development is not a program solely unfolding under genetic
control. It is a system exquisitely sensitive to specific experiences.

As all parents know, rolling over, reaching, crawling, standing,
and walking are significant events in the development of motor
control in infancy. Infants begin reaching for things between 4 and
5 months of age, but their manual dexterity leaves a lot to be desired.
As infants gain control over the hands and arms, they plan more
and more efficient actions. When anticipating contact with an object,
infants quickly adjust the trajectory of their arm(s) and modify their
hand shape depending on the location and properties of the object.
With greater control of their arms and hands, infants are able to use
tools. For example, when feeding using a spoon, there is a correct
way to pick up and orient a spoon. Holding it such that the food end
is toward the center of the body and such that the food stays on the
spoon allows for easy access to the mouth and success in feeding.
Around the middle of the first year, when infants begin eating solid
food, control of speed, movement, and orientation of the spoon rapidly come on line (Keen, 2011).

An even more sophisticated example comes from infants' carrying objects while locomoting. Crawling or walking brings infants
into self-propelled contact with distant objects. Infants also like to
share objects with other people, and often carry objects while crawling or walking. Both crawlers and walkers engage in any number
of strategies to carry objects (see Figure 2.11), and the more experiences infants have moving around, the more they carry objects
while moving. Surprisingly, walkers fall less when carrying objects
than not. Despite engaging in a more attention-demanding task –
walking *and* carrying – infants exercise greater balance control compared to when not carrying objects.

Although achievements in locomotion (i.e., from crawling to
cruising to walking) are expected as infants age, infants' abilities to
negotiate challenging motor tasks, such as descending a sloped surface or moving through an opening, are not automatic. Nonetheless,
infants are eventually adept at considering the properties of surfaces
and openings, such as the degree of slant or width of a doorway, and
explore different methods of getting around, such as crawling back-
ward or turning their body sideways, before settling on any specific
one (successful) mode.

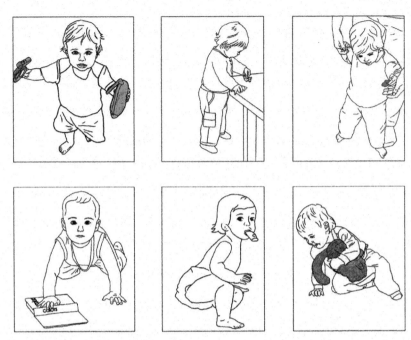

Figure 2.11 Different modes of carrying objects by crawlers and walkers. (From Karasik et al., 2012. Copyright © 2012 by the American Psychological Association. Reproduced with permission. The use of APA information does not imply endorsement by APA.)

Some infants of a given age might be crawlers, others walkers. Suppose you were to place one of each kind of baby at a precipice where the drop-offs were either small steps or steep cliffs as one study did (Kretch & Adolph, 2013). Experienced 12-month-old crawlers stop at the precipice and refuse to go over the cliff, but novice 12-month-old walkers will step over the cliff with abandon and need to be rescued from falling. With every new mode of getting around, infants must re-assess the conditions for safe locomotion. Each hour, the average toddler takes an estimated 1,200 steps and falls 16 times!

In the whole-child view of infant development, progress in one system, say walking, has implications for other systems. Unsurprisingly, motor development affects other domains of psychological growth. The advent of motor control more than just heralds cognitive development and social interaction – it instigates both. At a certain point, infants achieve control over their posture. A vertical posture soothes infants, enhances attention and alertness, stimulates goal-directedness and visual exploration which all together enrich cognition and social interaction. Grasping and reaching increase infants' appreciation of object properties, and different hand and arm movements reveal different object features. For example, poking an object with your finger tells you if it is hard or soft, tracing the edge of the object provides information about shape, and hefting an object reveals its weight. Infants learn about the object world from poking, tracing, and hefting. Moreover, 3½-month-old infants (called "pre-reachers") who explored objects by use of mittens outfitted with Velcro (so the objects stuck to their fingers and did not drop off) show advanced object perception relative to infants who did not have the same experience or who were merely shown objects (Figure 2.12; Libertus & Needham, 2010). Thus, the experience of exploring objects on one's own gives infants a head start in object exploration generally and enhances infants' understanding of interactions people have with objects.

The advent of crawling is even associated with improved memory: 9-month-old crawlers recalled an action they saw in one location when they were tested in the same or in a different location, whereas same-aged infants who were not yet crawlers recalled the

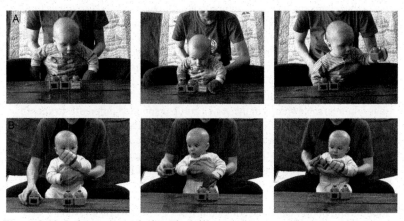

Figure 2.12 Infants provided with different object exploration experiences. (A) Infants wear mittens that stick to the objects and thus facilitate self-produced object exploration. (B) The objects do not stick to the mittens; thus, the parent must hold the object for the infant to explore visually. (From Libertus & Needham, 2010; reprinted from *Vision Research*, *50*(24), Libertus & Needham, Teach to reach: The effects of active vs. passive reaching experiences on action and perception, 2750–2757, 2010, with permission from Elsevier.)

action when tested in the same location but not when tested in a different location. Presumably, experience with self-locomotion affords infants opportunities to retrieve information across a range of contexts and leads to improved encoding or remembering information. As one research group noted, "travel broadens the mind" (Campos et al., 2000), and enlarging experiences may have long-term and diverse developmental consequences (Box 2.4).

Infant motor development further influences facets of parent–infant interaction. A baby first reaching deliberately, rolling over, crawling, standing upright, or walking occasions joy, photographs, and face-timing grandparents. These achievements also signal all sorts of changes at home, like "child proofing" (or moving dangerous items out of reach or installing locks on cupboards). More directly, moving infants can take an active role in how close or far away they wander from the parents, and interactions may

---

BOX 2.4   Set for Life? Motor Development and Reading

Is there a link between motor development and reading? A compelling example of the relation between infant motor development and child cognitive functioning comes from a Finnish study of the precursors of reading (Lyytinen et al., 2001). The Jyvaskyla Longitudinal Study of Dyslexia tracked children at risk for reading impairment and a comparison group of children without known risk from birth through 9 years of age. The researchers initially surveyed expectant families in and around the Finnish city of Jyvaskyla and eventually recruited 410 parents with suspected dyslexia and a matched group of normal volunteers. Newborns in the at-risk group responded differently to speech sounds by ERP, and by 6 months infants in the two groups displayed subtle but reliable differences in categorizing speech sounds and processing of non linguistic auditory stimuli. A fascinating twist emerged, however, when the researchers later considered motor development (Viholainen et al., 2002, 2006). At-risk children whose motor development was delayed during the first year of life had more limited vocabularies and shorter sentences at 18 and 24 months and poorer language competence at 3 and 5 years of age. At age 7, the at-risk children with slow motor development read more poorly than children in the control group, including children in the control group with slow motor development. However, children in the genetically at-risk group (those with dyslexic parents) with good motor development read as well as children in the control group! Because this study only looked at relations, we cannot conclude that slow motor development caused poor later reading. Instead, it is likely that one or more mechanism underlying good and poor readers also underlies motor development.

become more positive *and* more negative as infants achieve independence, but infants can now also get into potentially dangerous situations.

Infant motor development is nothing short of remarkable. Helpless neonates unable even to move from being placed on their backs become exhausting toddlers, locomoting helter-skelter around the house, in a very short year or two. A popular – if apocryphal – anecdote that circulates among parents holds that, at the height of his physical prowess, Jim Thorpe (the Olympian and professional football and baseball player who is often credited as the greatest athlete of the 20th century) was asked to do everything for 1 day that a toddler did, exactly the way the toddler did it. As the story goes, Thorpe gave up exhausted after a few hours, whereas the toddler continued blithely and incessantly about his business for the rest of the day. By studying infants, we are often reminded of just how complicated some seemingly simple behaviors are. As adults, we sit up and we walk automatically without a second thought, but watching a young baby's repeated failures to accomplish such simple feats forces us to reconsider just how much coordination of motor, orientation, posture, balance, and other skills is involved. We gain a new and deep appreciation of growing structure and function by studying their emergence and development in infancy.

SUMMARY

Physical and motor growth before birth and in the short span of infancy are impressive. Moreover, this growth supports extraordinary concurrent and future accomplishments like locomotion, language, and sociality. Genetics and experiences co-determine growth in infancy. Prenatal development is distinguished by identifiable stages and sensitive periods during which certain experiences are especially influential. Neurological developments occurring pre- and postnatally correspond to or underpin many observable trends that interest developmental scientists. Infants initially lack the capacity to modulate their own states of arousal and thus seem to shift erratically from one state to another. However, infants come to show consistent (if gross) cyclic organization of state. Neurological development underlies the emergence of organized patterns of sleeping and waking. Predictable changes in heart rate in response to various types of stimulation provide a powerful tool for assessing infants' states of development and general responsivity. In the CNS, intracellular and intercellular structure and function change dramatically over the first years of life as neurons are born, develop, and interconnect to permit increasingly efficient transmission of complex information. Neural plasticity is a hallmark of infancy. With increasing maturity, infants gain more and more control over their own movements, opening up their independent exploration of their world. Physical and motor development also provide models and metaphors for other spheres of infant growth and have implications for thinking, communicating, feeling, and relating domains of infant development.

THINKING

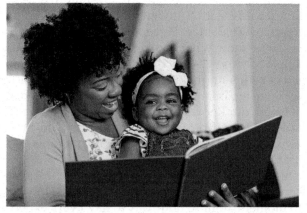

(Image courtesy of Shutterstock, copyright: pixelheadphoto digitalskillet/ Shutterstock.com.)

INTRODUCTION

Babies' brains grow and neurons connect with each other at an astonishing pace, but do infants *think*? Thinking entails many components from sensing and perceiving to learning and remembering to representing and interpreting. This chapter recounts infants' capacities in all these areas, and perhaps by the end of reading this chapter you will agree that infants definitely think.

DOI: 10.4324/9781003172802-3

Infants' number one job (besides eating and sleeping) is to come to know their physical and social worlds quickly, and thinking in all its forms lies at the heart of succeeding at that job. From passing observation, it is understandably hard to believe that anything like thinking is going on in the beginning or middle of infancy, but by the end of infancy, a brief 18 months later, it is equally hard to believe that anything but thinking must have been going on. How else could that "intake-sleep-output-repeat" system so speedily come to understand so much and make so many needs and wants so abundantly clear?

Sensing and perceiving constitute necessary first steps in experiencing and interpreting the world. Yet, the senses themselves need to develop. Happily, as developmental scientists have found, sensory development took full advantage of the 9 prenatal months to reach, not full-blown maturity, but an advanced stage of growth and adequate readiness to experience and interpret the world outside the womb. Sensing (seeing) is presumptive to perceiving (interpreting what is seen). Understanding babies' perceptions presents a formidable challenge: Perception is private. There is no way for one person to know what another person's perceptions are like. No two people can know what "blue" really is to the other. Sharing perceptions depends on making inferences from verbal reports or behaviors. However, infants are mute and motorically underdeveloped. As a result, our knowledge of infants' inner perceptual world is necessarily inferred from passing fragments (and little wonder that babies' caregivers constantly search for patterns to tell them what their LO is thinking).

What babies simply attend to is an important first step to sensing and perceiving. Furthermore, as infants experience the world, from moment to moment, hour to hour, day to day, every experience cannot be totally new, elsewise infants would not at all progress in their understanding of the physical and social worlds. Consequently, infants must be capable of learning and remembering, and this chapter describes some of the main ways developmental scientists have concluded that infants learn and remember. Finally, what do infants do with the knowledge they are accruing, however rudimentary that knowledge is. After all, that knowledge brings them to the end of infancy when they see and hear the world, perceive and remember faces, have learned scripts like eating, bath time, and sleeping, and even know some rules of elementary games.

Faithful to the whole-child view, infants apply all these sorts of thinking to communicating, feeling, and relating as will become clear in the next chapters. To begin to discuss infant thinking in all its forms, however, it is worthwhile to briefly rehearse those grand philosophical questions that stimulated widespread interest in infancy and infants' thinking in the first place.

SENSING AND PERCEIVING

Interest in infant sensation and perception was initiated by those philosophers we introduced in Chapter 1 who pondered the origins of knowledge and morality (because religion and firm belief in God was so pervasive in the intellectual traditions that revolved around those philosophical questions). About knowledge, extreme views were put forward by philosophical empiricists, who asserted that all intelligence comes through the senses and grows by way of experience, versus philosophical nativists, who reasoned that human beings must enter the world with rudimentary intelligence that helps to order and organize all that they experience. This knowledge debate as the dispute about right, had Biblical origins. If God created humankind in his image (Genesis 1:27), surely infants were both "knowledgeable" and "good." To speculate philosophically about the origins of mind and morals (or to prove one or the other position empirically) meant focusing attention on the beginning of life – infancy. What, if anything do infants know? And, are infants inherently good or evil?

Philosophical speculation and argument are indeterminate, depending on which advocate is the more erudite, articulate, or persuasive, and religion depends fundamentally on the "leap of faith." It was not until around the turn of the 20th century, when scientific experimentation was introduced into the study of sensation and perception, that the knowledge question began to yield enlightened (but still far from conclusive) answers. (Answers to the morals question may only be found in the mind of the believer.)

Scientific study provides information about the quality, limits, and capacities of sensations and perceptions. Determining how the senses function in infancy has permitted developmental scientists to glimpse the infant's world and revealed which features of the environment likely influence early development. Understanding sensation and perception in infancy is also valuable because it provides a starting point against which maturation and the effects of experience in development can be judged.

Consider momentarily a concrete example in one classic philosophical controversy. It concerns the ways infants come to perceive depth in space. Depth perception – seeing and knowing what is near and what is far – is crucial to determining the spatial layout of the environment, recognizing objects, and guiding motor action. Imagine, for a moment, if you could not see depth. How would you know if it was safe to step down a stair? When would you know if you were about to bang into a wall? Could you reach for that cup of coffee without knocking it over? Early philosophers were puzzled by the fact that we immediately perceive the world as three-dimensional (3D) and easily negotiate our way through a room on the basis of 3D cues. But think about how that visual information is processed, recalling that three dimensionality begins as two dimensions on the surface of the flat retina at the back of the eye. How would an infant ever know depth or the three dimensions of space? What began as a hotly contested philosophical dispute that spanned the 17th to 19th centuries finally yielded to developmental science experimentation in the 20th century.

As you might surmise by now, a tennis match of opinion unfolded over nearly three centuries. An early serve offered by nativist Descartes (whom we met in Chapter 1) asserted infants perceive depth in visual space as an inborn God-given ability based on the fact that they have two eyes, separated in space, that give two different perspectives on the world. English empiricist George Berkeley (1685–1753) counterargued that no such complex knowledge could be present at birth, but rather infants learn about depth through feedback from their tactile and motor experience. Infants associate "near" with the small amount they have to move their arms when reaching for close objects and "far" with the greater amount when reaching for objects at a distance. German nativist Immanuel Kant (1724–1804), in turn, retorted that the human mind could never solely rely on experience for such rich meaning (depth perception emerges too early in life to be based on extensive experience and learning), but the mind innately organizes sensations into meaningful perceptions of depth. To which German empiricist Hermann Helmholtz (1821–1894) argued back that it is uneconomical to assume mechanisms of innate perception, especially when innate sensations are likely overruled by the more accurate understandings obtained through actual experience. Whether any one of these philosophers ever consulted a baby first-hand (other perhaps than their own) is unknown.

And so debate went until experimental study finally replaced philosophical speculation. In fact, experimental psychology, which only came into its own in the 20th century, was specifically organized to address just such questions. We return to the developmental science contribution to the resolution of this depth perception puzzle later in this chapter. First, however, we need to know some things about development of the sensory systems in infants.

SENSING AND PERCEIVING IN INFANCY

The principal way we get information from the environment is through our senses: sight, hearing, smell, taste, and touch. All senses develop and begin to function before birth. By the second trimester, the eye and visual system, the ear and auditory system, the nose and olfactory system, the tongue and gustatory system, and the skin and somatosensory system are essentially mature structurally, although their levels of functional competence lag behind. Two generalizations about the development of the sensory systems in infancy are well established. First, maturation within systems tends to occur peripherally (at the sense organ) before it occurs centrally (in the brain). So, for example, the eye is structurally developed and functions before the visual cortex does. Second, different senses achieve structural and functional maturity at different times: for example, touch then hearing then vision. This staggered developmental schedule appears to permit development to concentrate on reaching high levels of maturity one at a time.

TASTE AND SMELL

Newborn babies can discriminate among sensory qualities that signify different tastes and smells, and they even prefer certain tastes and smells to others (Figure 1.7). Elements of foods that mothers eat can be found in the amniotic fluid surrounding fetuses, and fetuses develop flavor preferences that last into childhood and adulthood. Neonates also distinguish odors placed on cotton swabs held beneath their nose. In Chapter 1, we described how newborns respond in qualitatively different ways to different food odors: Butter and banana odors elicit positive expressions; vanilla, either positive or indifferent expressions; a fishy odor, some rejection; and the odor of rotten eggs, unanimous rejection.

An odor that is particularly appealing to young infants and learned very quickly is that of their mother. Porter and colleagues (1988) systematically compared olfactory recognition of mother, father, and stranger by breastfed and bottle-fed infants only 2 weeks after birth. Babies were exposed to pairs of gauze pads worn by these different adults in the underarm area on the previous night, and babies' duration of orienting to the different pads was recorded. Only breastfeeding infants oriented preferentially to their own mother's scent, thereby giving evidence that they discriminate and prefer their mother to others. Infants did not recognize their fathers preferentially, and bottle-fed infants did not recognize their mothers by her odor at this early age. The ability to recognize mothers very early in life by olfactory information alone might play an important role in the early mother–infant relationship, at least for breast fed infants. All infants have other cues they use to recognize important people, such as their face and the sound of their voice.

SEEING

The eye develops rapidly in the first and second trimesters of gestation, although neural pathways in the brain that support vision continue to develop well into postnatal life. Infants' ability to see fine detail is limited, and thus newborns cannot clearly see most objects or people beyond 18 inches (45 cm) away. As such, newborns could be described as legally blind. When considering the different developmental trajectories of vision and the other senses, it is important to keep in mind that other senses can be and are stimulated before birth, whereas full visual stimulation is only experienced after birth. To the extent that experience influences development, vision is at a disadvantage.

To return now to the question of depth perception, three lines of research were pursued that illustrate how questions about the origins of perceiving depth were eventually addressed experimentally (Arterberry & Kellman, 2016). No one line provides definitive information, but the three together converge to draw a more convincing picture of infant's appreciation of depth in space.

The starting point for one line of research was an observation purportedly made by Eleanor J. Gibson (1910–2002), a U.S. developmental scientist, while on vacation with her family at the Grand Canyon. Her young child began crawling perilously close to the edge. Her husband, U.S. perceptual psychologist James J. Gibson (1904–1979), said that there was no reason to worry because there was plenty of visual information alerting the child to the cliff (which is true, as you will see below). Yet, Eleanor Gibson still moved the child away from danger, musing that young infants and toddlers are notoriously prone to falls. It may be in this moment the first experimental question about the development of depth perception was asked. What information do babies use to perceive depth and when?

In the best tradition of developmental scientists, Gibson and her colleague Walk (1960) promptly began to investigate depth perception in infants using a **visual cliff** (Figure 3.1). One side of the cliff

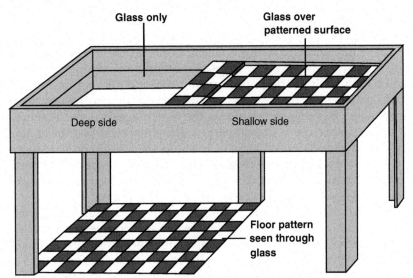

Figure 3.1 The visual cliff. There is glass on both sides, but on one side there is a deep space between the glass and the checkered floor whereas on the other shallow side the checks are right under the glass. Infants are placed on the centerboard and observed regarding whether they are willing to cross the deep side. (From Gibson & Walk, 1960; reproduced with permission.)

shows the baby an illusory drop, but the other side does not. Few infants between 6 and 14 months of age crawled across the deep side when their mothers called them. These results suggest that depth perception must be present in infants as young as 6 months of age. Well, you might argue, by 6 months children may already have had plenty of experience perceiving depth. Recall from Chapter 1 that heart rate can be used to indicate attention. Babies as young as 2 months of age show a decrease in heart rate when exposed to the deep as opposed to the shallow side of the visual cliff, indicating increased attention to depth. Thus, babies give evidence that they perceive depth long before they crawl or walk (but still show little fear of depth). Perhaps the wariness of drop offs shown by infants results, not from actual experience with falls, but from the anxiety parents display when their infants approach a drop off. Infants regularly look to their parents and use their parents' emotional cues to interpret ambiguous events (called **social referencing**, discussed in Chapter 6).

Visual cliff experiments represent one way to explore infants' capacity to perceive depth. In actuality, different types of stimulus information help to specify depth. Both Descartes and Kant were on to something because our two eyes do receive slightly different images of the visual world (to see for yourself, close one eye and look straight ahead; now open that eye and close the other; the scene jumps a bit as you continue alternating opening and closing each eye), and differences between the two images are a proven cue for depth. Infants are sensitive to this disparity between the two images around 4 months of age. Another cue is the convergence angle of the two eyes, that is how much our eyes need to rotate toward each other in order to focus on an object: a lot for very close objects, hardly at all for distant ones. Infants 3 months, and perhaps younger, converge their eyes when an object approaches and diverge their eyes when it recedes.

But wait; there are more cues that infants and adults might use for perceiving depth. A second line of research focuses on so-called pictorial depth cues. Static monocular cues (meaning they are available to a stationary observer who only needs one eye to use them) to depth are well known and often referred to as pictorial depth cues because artists as far back as Leonardo da Vinci in the Renaissance used them to give the illusion of depth to a flat painting. One such cue is linear perspective, where two lines known to be parallel in real life (like railroad tracks) are seen to converge with distance. Texture elements that are small in size or tightly knit cue closeness, and those large in size or loosely knit cue distance. Interposition occurs when contours of one object partially block another object from view; the first object is perceived to be closer than the second. Infants between 5 and 7 months of age are sensitive to all these pictorial cues.

A third line of research focuses on cues involving motion, either of the objects or of the observer. These dynamic cues to depth include looming, as when an object is coming directly toward us, its image on our retina expands. In this situation, we normally perceive the object as getting closer (and move to avoid the impending collision). Babies as young as 1 month consistently blink at approaching objects (even on a screen so that air turbulence is not a cue).

In summary, experiments demonstrate that infants are sensitive to different types of depth information at different ages, with motion cues emerging earliest, ocular cues (such as convergence and disparity) emerging next, and pictorial depth cues emerging last. Circling back to philosophy, neither nativists nor empiricists might ever claim a final triumph. No matter how early in life depth perception can be demonstrated, the ability still rests on some experience, and no matter how late depth perception emerges, it can never be proved that only experience has mattered.

The story of depth perception illustrates the philosophy-to-science history of infants' beginning understanding of the world. Similar questions have been asked about infants' rudimentary perceptions of form, orientation, and motion. When and how well do infants first see forms? Do they see forms as a unit (as a triangle) or as individual elements (lines and angles and surfaces)? Of course, some theorists, such as Wolfgang Köhler (1887–1967), a German psychologist, proposed that the perception of whole forms is innate, whereas other theorists, such as the Canadian psychologist Donald Hebb (1904–1985), proposed that perception of whole forms is built up from perceptions of individual elements – lines and angles and surfaces. Today, scholars in the neo-nativist school have forsaken Biblical reasoning in favor of evolutionary biology. From an evolutionary biological perspective, the visual system adapted to perceive movement because doing so carries distinct survival advantages: Things that move bring protection, nutrition, danger, and opportunities for exploration. Suffice it to say that questions about form, orientation, and motion perception have likewise been mired in philosophical debates but yielded scientific headway. Through systematic application of the methods described in Chapter 1, developmental scientists have learned in broad outline that infants perceive forms, are aware of variation in orientation, and discern different kinds of motion, but that the details and nuances of the first origins and developmental trajectories of these infant perceptual abilities still elude final judgment.

Our world is filled with 3D objects, and they are specified in many ways, as by their orientation, location, and motion. Have a look at your nearby coffee mug. If you place it on the table and then walk to the other side of the table, it may look different. For example, the handle might not be visible, or if it is visible the handle's shape might appear to be different from when you saw it earlier. The logo on the front of the cup might not match the logo on the back of the cup. However, you have no trouble recognizing your cup. You might remember what the back of the cup looks like from previous experience, and you know that you just walked to the other side of the table. However, it is unlikely that you have seen and remember each and every possible variation of the cup in space. More likely, you rely on some key principles of perception. Solid objects do not change, even when our viewpoints of them do. Being able to recognize an object from different perspectives is an important step to experiencing a stable perceptual environment. **Viewpoint invariance** entails understanding that an object viewed from different viewpoints is still the same object. Infants appear to possess viewpoint invariance. In one study, 5-month-olds were habituated

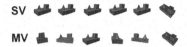

Figure 3.2 Stimuli used to test infants' recognition of an object across multiple viewpoints. Infants in the SV group saw the Same View of the object during the habituation phase. In contrast, infants in the MV group saw Multiple Views. At test, the same object was presented in a different orientation. (From Mash et al., 2007; reproduced with permission from Wiley.)

to a simple object (one they had never seen before) either by a series of images depicting a single view of the object or by a series depicting different views of the object around its vertical axis (Mash et al., 2007; Figure 3.2). Infants in the single view group failed to recognize the same object when it was inverted, but infants in the group who saw multiple views successfully recognized the object when it was inverted. Thus, babies in the first year of life perceive different views of the same 3D object as exactly that – views from the same object.

In the whole-child perspective, each ability an infant commands is associated with or feeds into another ability. For example, perceiving movement is important to **figural coherence**, perceptually grouping elements of an object that have invariant spatial relations to one another. A compelling example of figural coherence is the so-called **point-light display** (PLD). Suppose you attach Christmas lights to each joint on the body of one person (Figure 3.3A), and you attach the same number of lights randomly around the body of a second person (Figure 3.3B). Now turn on the lights, and in the dark film the two people walking so that all that is filmed are the moving lights. It takes adults two-tenths of a second to identify Figure 3.3A as a human being, whereas Figure 3.3B makes no sense as anything (and static displays of the same information are equally un interpretable). Infants do not perceive Figure 3.3A as unrelated swarms of randomly moving dots, nor do they focus on the motion paths of individual lights. Rather, infants are sensitive to the overall coherence of the figure based on its biomechanical motion, and as young as 6 months of age appear to perceive displays such as Figure 3.3A to depict a solid object. Somewhat older infants even categorize motion patterns as specific to different emotions and different sexes.

Patterns and objects in the environment vary in terms of spatial dimensions that help specify, identify, and distinguish them. They

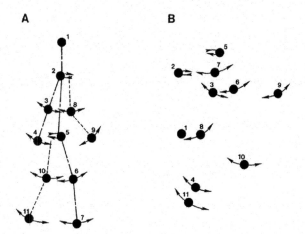

Figure 3.3 (A) An array of 11-point lights attached to the head and joints of a walking person: The head and right side of the body are numbered 1 through 7, and the numbers 8 through 11 mark those of the body's left side. The motion vectors drawn through each point light represent the perceived relative motions within the figure. (B) An anomalous walker identical to A except that the relative locations of the point lights have been scrambled as shown. (Correspondingly numbered point lights have the same absolute motions.) (Reprinted from *Journal of Experimental Child Psychology*, 37(2), Bertenthal et al., 1984, Infant sensitivity to figural coherence in biomechanical motions, 213–230, with permission from Elsevier.)

are also perceived as having color. Color is aesthetically attractive. Spoiler alert: Infants see colors and seem to do so, not perfectly, but pretty well. Color vision harbors three dimensions: **hue** is the term we most closely associate with color (red, yellow, etc.), but colors also have **brightness** (how luminant a color is: bright red versus dark red) and **saturation** (how vivid the color is: cadmium red versus pink). Because every color we see has some hue, brightness, and saturation, it has been estimated that the human eye can distinguish about 10 million different colors. But, if we show a baby a red and a green circle, and the baby looks more at one than the other, we do not really know if the baby is preferring the red hue over the green hue or the brighter color or the more saturated color. As a consequence, understanding infant color vision needs to take all three dimensions into consideration simultaneously. That is, brightness and saturation need to be controlled to find out if infants discriminate, prefer, and organize hue alone.

To simplify the discussion and because it may be the most interesting of the three dimensions, we focus on just hue. Developmental scientists were able to discover that, across a broad range of conditions, infants successfully discriminate blue, green, yellow, and red by 3 months of age and prefer (look longer at) red and blue than green and yellow. But there is more to color perception than just perceiving individual hues. Adults perceive that the color spectrum is organized into qualitative **categories of hue**: bright reds and dark reds, cadmium and pinks are all still "red" and different from blues, greens, and yellows. The infant's color space is similarly organized at least by 4 months of age (Bornstein, 2007).

HEARING

Much less is known about how infants hear than about how they see, even though hearing is of major importance to infants. Make a sudden loud noise and even a neonate will startle. The auditory system is highly developed, if not yet fully mature, at the time of birth. Although the stomach and uterine wall insulate sounds before birth, neonates soon after birth prefer the sound of their mother's voice, indicating that fetuses hear sounds coming from outside of the uterus, including mother's heartbeat and her voice (but there is no evidence that playing fetuses Mozart will make a difference to their musicality).

Human speech is a complex interplay of different sound **frequencies** (pitch) at different **amplitudes** (loudness) distributed over time. Infancy researchers have focused principally on the way babies respond to complex sounds that specify human speech. Young babies attend selectively to and imitate human over nonhuman sounds, and parents conveniently and unthinkingly adjust their speech in many ways to accommodate their infants' sensitivities. **Infant-directed speech** (IDS) simplifies normal adult-directed speech in sound patterns, words used, grammatical complexity, and gesture. IDS has higher pitch, exaggerated intonation, a sing-song rhythm, shorter utterances, and more repetitions. Think about how you greet a baby (or your pet) – "Hel-LO BA-By!" IDS is also nearly universal across cultures.

From all the possible speech sounds that can be produced (**phonetics**), each language uses only a subset of sounds to create meaning (**phonemics**) used in speech. For example, some languages use sounds like "ma" or "pa" (e.g., English), whereas others use "clicks" (e.g., African Bantu). Of course, different people say "ma" or "pa" in different ways (think of New Englanders in the

U.S. versus Australians), and even the same person likely enunciates "ma" or "pa" in different ways at different times. **Categorical perception** involves treating as similar otherwise discriminable stimuli and treating as different other qualitatively distinct stimuli. For example, babies only 1 month old treat variations in sounds like "ma" as similar and different from variations in sounds like "pa." Indeed, infants in the first 6 months distinguish many such sound contrasts.

The demonstration of such a hearing ability so early in life may seem to support nativists, but it does not rule out a role for nurture. It could be that the prenatal experience of hearing sounds induces or tunes fetuses' and infants' discrimination abilities. Also, babies have a full postnatal month of hearing "ma"s and "pa"s ("Honey, look at mama! Sweetheart, see what papa is doing!"). However, developmental scientists have learned that infants distinguish many sound contrasts even in languages they have never heard. One investigator has called babies "citizens of the world" because they start life being able to distinguish sounds in many languages, even sounds not in their own language. Alas, in the absence of continuing exposure to sounds not in their language, babies eventually lose the ability to hear many differences. By contrast, infants reared in multilingual environments continue to possess those abilities. It is as though babies arrive with a brand-new auditory system capable of learning whatever language they hear, but they need to be exposed to a language to maintain and further develop language.

INTEGRATING SENSATION, PERCEPTION, AND ACTION

We briefly discussed the senses as though they are separate, but in everyday life the senses do not behave separately. Information coming into our senses is coordinated. When we are at the beach, we see the waves, hear the surf, smell the salt air, touch the sand, feel the sun on our skin, and so forth. Likewise, information obtained from the senses is often coordinated from very early in life.

Curiously, however, developmental scientists (like their philosophical forebears) do not really know whether sensations are initially integrated and then differentiate with development or sensations are initially fragmented and integrate with development. Maybe newborns' senses are unified at birth in that they perceive something loud, something bright, or something painful to touch all at the same moment and as high on a single dimension of intensity and only come to distinguish loudness from brightness from painfulness with time. A strong view of this perspective is that very young babies may not know whether they are hearing or seeing or feeling something. A contrasting school of thought (of course!) argues that the processes involved in integrating information are complicated, that very young babies are unable to integrate information from the different senses, and that the ability to coordinate input across senses develops over the first years of life through coordinated experience. At the moment, integrationists appear to have the day. Objects and events are specified along dimensions of information, and infants respond to objects and events, regardless of sensory modality. For example, newborn infants visually recognize objects that they previously explored by touch (Sann & Streri, 2008).

Moreover, perception and action go together. We move in order to perceive (we move our eyes, our head, and our limbs), and as a result of perceiving we might move (reach to grasp an object or avoid something noxious). The two go hand in hand; perceiving leads to acting and acting leads to perceiving. Young infants turn their head toward a sound source to visually inspect the source. Visually tracking extends to reaching: Infants reach and grasp moving objects. Watch babies look and then reach out and grasp a ball; before even touching the ball, babies prepare for the grasp by modifying their hand shape based on visual information. Infants learn about shape, substance, and other object properties by coordinated and integrated exploring. Even blind infants manually explore: They shake, bang, mouth, and finger objects similarly to sighted infants.

Even though the senses are remarkably developed at birth, perceptual experience is still critical to ensure normal psychological growth and development. As the foregoing example about speech sounds attests, nature and nurture work hand-in-glove. The infant nervous system is wired to be sensitive to experience and specific experience further shapes the sensitivity of the nervous system. Frankly, evolution could not have designed a better or more flexible solution. In the whole-child perspective, motor and perceptual experience matter to cognitive and social development, as the "sticky mittens" study also reveals (Figure 2.12).

Two more examples of the power of experience on development will bring home this lesson. As will be discussed in Chapter 4 on Communicating, at some point in the first year of life infants (even deaf infants) begin to babble. Very quickly, however, their babbling becomes specialized to the target language they hear and will eventually speak. One cross-cultural investigation by

Boysson-Bardies and colleagues (1984) recorded the babbling of 6-, 8-, and 10-month-old infants from different Parisian French, Hong Kong Cantonese, and Algiers Arabic language backgrounds and then played the recordings of those different babbles to French, Hong Kong, and Algerian adults asking them to identify which babbles came from infants from their own linguistic community. People from the three countries could do so successfully. This result shows that the specific sound characteristics of the target language young infants heard quickly shaped their babbling production.

Reciprocally, missing out on experience is equivalently telling on development. Cataracts cloud the lens of the eye and diminish vision. Many elderly people develop cataracts, and the treatment is surgical removal of the old clouded lens and insertion of a new clear lens. On occasion, infants are born with a cataract in one or both eyes. Infants who have two cataracts are deprived of binocular stimulation from birth. Tests of visual acuity (Box 3.1) administered within minutes of initial insertion of new lenses reveal modest but reliable improvements in infant visual acuity after just 1 hour of focused visual input. Tested years later, however, infants who had cataracts display some impaired perceptions. Notably, they have difficulty discriminating internal features of faces (eyes, nose, mouth), but can still discriminate emotional expressions. The fact that some abilities are affected and others spared suggests that specific brain regions underlie these areas and that some functions more readily recover after deprivation.

BOX 3.1   How Well Do Infants See You?

This is really a two-part question. Part 1 is how well infants see. Part 2 is how well they see faces.

PART 1

Robert Fantz (1925–1981), a U.S. developmental scientist, originated a preference technique to study **visual acuity**, or how well infants see fine detail (like going to the optometrist). Fantz and colleagues (1962) showed babies pairs of patterns. One member of the pair was always gray, and the other was a set of black-and-white stripes that varied systematically in width. (The two patterns were also always matched in overall brightness.) Infants prefer to look at heterogeneous rather than homogeneous patterns, so the stripe width that failed to evoke a preference (longer looking) was taken as the boundary of babys' ability to distinguish stripes from solid gray. Figure 3.4 shows an infant being tested for visual acuity this way, and Figures 3.5B and C provide a concrete idea of just how well young babies actually see compared to adults (Figure 3.5A). By this measure, infants show a remarkable development in visual acuity between 2 weeks and 5 months of age. In the 50 years since Fantz's original study, techniques for measuring infant visual acuity have grown in sophistication, but the results continue to agree with his initial findings. Visual acuity is relatively poor in newborns, but it improves rapidly and, by about 6 months of age, is almost the same as that of normal adults. This procedure has been adapted so that infant acuity can be assessed in a pediatrician's office and, if necessary, babies can be fitted with glasses.

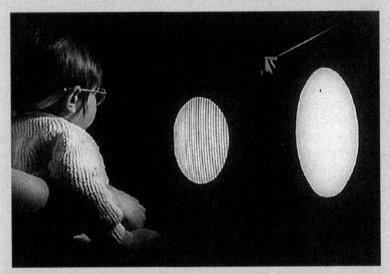

Figure 3.4 An infant's visual acuity being tested. (Courtesy of J. Atkinson and O. Braddock.)

PART 2

Infants of all ages are very attracted to faces. Unknown, however, is whether this attraction is based on an innate, species-specific predisposition to attend to faces (Johnson & Hannon, 2015) or is based on the fact that faces have visual properties that attract infants' attention, such as areas of high contrast and movement (Simion & Giorgio, 2015). At first, experiments with two-dimensional (2D) stimuli (photographs of faces) suggested that the basis for infants' attraction was the presence of contrasts in facial configurations. However, when 2D stimuli in a normal face pattern, a scrambled face pattern, and a blank stimulus are moved slowly in an arc-like path, newborns look at and track the normal face pattern significantly more than the other two stimuli suggesting an inborn preference for face-like stimuli (Johnson et al., 1991). We now know that, yes, faces have visual features, such as symmetry and high contrast, that attract infant attention and that these features may not be specific to faces, but at the same time there are cortical and subcortical mechanisms present at birth that with time will become specialized for face processing. As babies grow (and improve in their acuity), so does their face perception. For example, internal features of faces become more prominent as infants see finer details. Moreover, 5-month-old infants can discriminate between a face with typical spacing of the eyes and mouth from a face with exaggerated spacing between features, and they recognize faces across different emotional expressions. By 7–8 months, infants recognize the same face across different viewpoints.

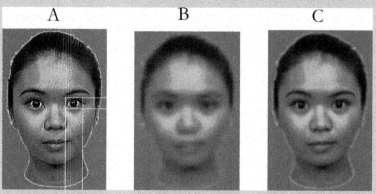

Figure 3.5 The faces show how they might appear to: (A) adults; (B) a newborn; and (C) a 4-month-old infant. (From Farroni et al., 2002, copyright (2002) National Academy of Sciences; reproduced with permission.)

COGNITION IN INFANCY

Infants' active mental life begins with sensing and perceiving but proceeds rapidly to more complex learning, developing new ideas, and remembering. Developmental scientists group these several abilities under the rubric of **cognition**. Infant cognition itself generates a series of compelling and puzzling questions. If we cannot ask infants, what is infant cognition anyway, how can it be measured, and what do infants learn? Consider all the people you know. They differ in how smart they are, how verbal they are, and how skilled they are. Do infants differ from one another in their mental abilities?

To develop our mental abilities, we attend formal school as well as gather life experiences. Where do infants begin in this process?

Infants' mental life is not divorced from their sensations and perceptions, but cognition builds on sensations and perceptions both directly and in terms of general principles. Consider for a moment what kind of mental life you yourself might engineer for the human infant. Certainly, you would not want to fix the infant's cognitive abilities in advance of any actual experience. It would be short sighted and counterproductive to disregard the possible beneficial effects of experience because cognitive skills naturally include the ability to adapt successfully to the surrounding and effective environment. By the same token, however, you would not want to leave mental development wholly to experience. Not all experience is optimal, and it is hardly infants' fault or responsibility to be condemned for life by chance deprivations of early experience. In fact, both criteria appear to have been met in the evolution of the development of infant cognition. As with their perceptions, infants are biologically prepared to learn and grow mentally from experiences provided by their physical and social ecologies. Keep these design criteria in mind as this discussion about cognition in infancy proceeds.

Some of what has been learned about infant cognition concerns what generally infants know, what they acquire, and how what they know guides their behavior. Our other understanding of infant cognition focuses on the growth of infants' mental life as specific individual differences among infants. For example, some infants habituate quickly, whereas others the same age habituate slowly. These two lines of thought about infant cognition – the general and the specific – complement one another.

PIAGET

Piaget watched closely as his own three children grew in infancy between 1925 and 1932, and he made note of the enormous progress each child made during their first 2 years of life. On that basis, he published a compilation of his observations and informal experiments (Piaget, 1952). Piaget (like his forebears) was initially motivated by a desire to resolve the nature-nurture debate about the origins of knowledge. However, Piaget believed neither nativist nor empiricist accounts. Rather, Piaget's novel solution was that infants construct or build knowledge based on their own motor activity and interactions in the world.

In newborns, many motor activities can be used to acquire or process information in the environment; sucking, grasping, looking, hearing, and tasting are examples. According to Piaget, knowledge begins to develop as the elaboration of simple behaviors present in the newborn. Motor activities dominate infancy, but eventually they are replaced with mental activities. For Piaget, infant cognition is not static; rather, infants create, respond to, and adjust to an ever-changing world. Infant mental development is also self-modifying, and Piaget developed two powerful concepts to explain how such modifications – essentially cognitive growth – comes about. Piaget trained as a biologist and conceived of cognitive growth (like all biological change) as **adaptation**, the fundamental process whereby motor and mental activity may be altered through experience. In his view, adaptation is accomplished by two complementary processes – **assimilation** and **accommodation**. When information can be incorporated into the existing way of acting or thinking, the information is said to be assimilated. Assimilation is a conservative process because the infant only incorporates new information and does not change an existing way of thinking or acting on the world. At times, however, existing motor or mental activity cannot success-fully assimilate new information. In this case, one of two things can happen. Either the infant can fail to assimilate and simply move on to another activity, or the infant can change to process new informa-tion. Modifying existing motor or mental activity to a new situation is accommodation. Importantly, children actively change to better adapt to their environment. Assimilation and accommodation con-stantly co-occur so that infants' minds come to match and under-stand reality more and more closely. In everyday life, the balance between assimilation and accommodation shifts, giving temporary pre-eminence to one or the other process depending on what infants are doing. For example, in pretend play reality can be interpreted in any way one wishes so assimilation predominates; during imitation the actions of the child change to match targets as closely as possible so accommodation predominates.

Piaget's theory of infant cognitive development stresses how the infant slowly and in stages progresses from egocentrism, infants' understanding of the world in terms of their own motor activity, to times when they begin to notice and focus on events in the out-side world and appreciate relations among objects outside them-selves. For Piaget, this achievement constituted the emergence of **mental representation**. For example, infants can now imagine the whereabouts of an invisible object for the first time, and infants are now also able to imitate people even in their absence. According to Piaget, attaining mental representation is made possible by many slow accommodations across the first 18 to 24 months of life.

Other developmental scientists have taken issue with Piaget's formulations, assumptions, and observations. Grounding all knowledge in motor activity mistakenly ignores the vital contributions of sensory and perceptual activity to representation and knowledge. A tragic natural experiment showed this to be the case. In the 1960s, some pregnant women took the drug thalidomide to combat nausea and morning sickness. If ingested in the first trimester, it turned out that thalidomide interfered with fetal limb differentiation, so that babies were born limbless. Despite the absence of normal sensorimotor experience through their infancy, affected children developed a normal cognitive life. It has also been shown that infants' capacity for perceiving and representing the physical world is much better developed than Piaget ever thought. As reviewed in Chapter 1, the fact that young infants habituate means that they represent information mentally. Very young infants respond to an adult modeling simple mouth movements – tongue protrusion, mouth opening, and lip pursing – by imitating those actions (Figure 3.6). Imitation requires representational abilities.

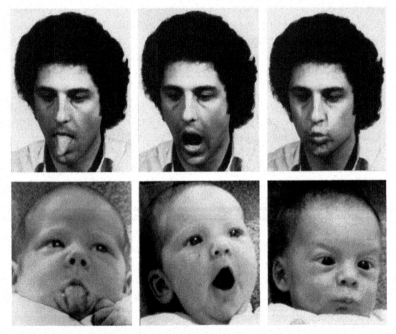

Figure 3.6 Two- to 3-week-old infants imitating. (Copyright © 1977 American Psychological Association. From Meltzoff & Moore, 1977; reproduced with permission.)

LEARNING

Piaget's is not the only or even the most prominent view of infant cognition today, even if it was novel if not revolutionary. Alternative learning and information-processing perspectives interpret infant cognition in terms of the acquisition of associations and the application of processing mechanisms to bring information from the external environment into the internal cognitive system. Like Piaget's theory, these theories propose rules that apply to all infants. For example, the laws of learning (like operant conditioning discussed in Chapter 1) are presumably universal and followed by all individuals and all species. Unlike Piaget's emphasis on normative development that applies to all infants, these two alternative approaches concentrate on individual differences in cognitive functioning. Learning and information processing are believed to account for the infant's slow but steady acquisition of knowledge about the world. Both mechanisms also reflect underlying brain plasticity and change.

There are three main kinds of learning, and each reflects the acquisition of some kind of association. **Classical conditioning** capitalizes on the existence of stimulus–response relations built into the organism, as when a loud sound elicits an eye blink. The loud sound is called the unconditioned stimulus (UCS; because it elicits a response in the absence of any learning or conditioning), and the response it gives rise to (the eye blink in this illustration) is called the unconditioned response (UCR). In classical conditioning, a conditioned stimulus (CS), a stimulus that is initially neutral and does not elicit the response, is paired with a UCS. Let's call an odor of vanilla the CS, and pair it with that loud sound (the UCS). After repeated pairings of the odor CS with the sound UCS, the odor CS takes on properties of the sound UCS and elicits an eye blink, the conditioned response (CR), like the UCR. That is, learning by association takes place. The famous example comes from the Russian physiologist Ivan Pavolv's (1849–1936) experiments with dogs, which learned to CR salivate to a CS bell that was paired with UCS food that naturally caused UCR salivation. Even newborns learn to make such associations and subsequently make use of what they have learned. For example, a UCR eye blink in newborns to a UCS air puff directed at the infants' eyelid was paired with a CS tone. Infants so conditioned made more anticipatory eye blinks when only the tone was presented than infants in a control group, in which the tones and puffs were presented at random. Does classical conditioning happen in real life? Suppose an infant was nipped at by a barking dog in the house. The nip (UCS) gives rise to a pain (UCR) that is paired with barking (CS). Voila!

Fear of dogs (CR). As we learn in Chapter 5, Watson (the empiricist from Chapter 1) appealed to classical conditioning to account for different infant emotions.

Operant conditioning involves associations between an action and the consequence of that action. Actions that are positively reinforced (rewarded in some way) are more likely to be repeated in the future, whereas actions that are negatively reinforced (punished in some way) are less likely to be repeated. Again, newborns only 1–4 days of age can be operantly conditioned, as shown when human speech and complex non speech were presented to babies contingent on their rate of sucking a blind nipple attached to a computer that generated a sound. In this experiment, infants could maintain hearing speech or non speech if they sucked faster. Most infants sucked so that they could continue to hear speech. The mobile paradigm described in Chapter 1 also relies on operant conditioning (Figure 1.8). Does operant conditioning happen in real life? Babies are interested in and pay attention to certain sounds and music; the two are reinforcing. Play *Baby Shark* for an infant (if you dare) and see if the infant does not want to watch the video more and more!

Observation combined with **imitation** is a third and particularly efficient way to learn – just by watching or listening. Newborns only days of age imitate, maybe not everything, but some things they can (like sticking out a tongue or opening a mouth; Figure 3.6). Imitation only grows in power as infancy proceeds. Infants quickly learn some straightforward concepts by imitation, such as tool use. Infants pick up on certain actions that others do, such as how to use a spoon, and soon want to do it for themselves. Infants also learn about more sophisticated associations by observation, such as cause and effect between physical objects and between people as, for example, watching a human press a button on a box that turns on a light in the box and causes another box to dispense a marble. Infants 24 months of age learn the connection between the human's actions and its effects by watching, but they do not make the connection when the effects happen without human action (Meltzoff et al., 2012).

Of course, there are limits to infant learning. Older infants learn faster than younger infants. Learning takes place most readily and efficiently during periods of quiet alertness, and not surprisingly infants who are drowsy or crying learn less. What is to be learned also matters. Classical conditioning is not established with every kind of stimulus, and not every behavior can be strengthened through operant reinforcement, just as not every act can be imitated. Infants must be able to perceive the stimulus and be physically capable of the response demanded. Appreciating these limits is important for three reasons: For what they tell us about learning, about infancy, and about what parents can and should expect of their infants' mental development (and parents' expectations of their infants are highly significant to infant development, as will be covered in Chapter 6). Finally, the fact that infants can learn does not guarantee that they always make use of all these learning devices in their daily life. This is a good example of the distinction between competence (being able to do a thing) and performance (actually doing the thing).

The ways babies learn are complemented by how babies simply regard the world and process information about it. The phenomenon developmental scientists call **information processing** tells us about the activities infants use in representing and manipulating information mentally. As a reminder, in Chapter 1 we described how infants will typically orient and attend to a novel stimulus, but if that stimulus is repeated or remains available to view, infants' attention usually wanes. Habituation is the decline in responding to a stimulus that is presented repeatedly or continuously. If infants are then shown both the familiar and a new stimulus after habituation, they will tend to look at the familiar stimulus less and at the novel stimulus more called novelty responsiveness. It stands to reason that habituation and novelty responsiveness reflect (at least) two component processes – the construction of a mental representation of the stimulus (a memory) and the continuing comparison between the repeated stimulus and that mental representation. Otherwise, first, the repeated stimulus would be responded to as new on each successive presentation and, second, there would be no reason that the two stimuli would be regarded as different after habituation. Thus, infants' disinterest in the now familiar stimulus presumably indicates that they have learned and remembered something about the repeated stimulus. That is, infants have processed stimulus information.

And, as Chapter 1 suggested, just like adults some infants learn or process stimulus information more quickly, efficiently, or completely than others. These individual differences tell us about infants' present and future mental life. For example, other things being equal, some infants habituate to an image, say of an animal, in seconds, whereas others may take minutes. Moreover, an infant is likely to habituate in approximately the same way on different occasions; that is, a baby's style of processing information is relatively consistent and so indicative of something constant about the baby. Likewise, infants vary in their ability to remember stimuli. These processing and memory indices predict children's performance on a variety of mental tasks as long as 14 years later (Box 3.2).

BOX 3.2   Set for Life? Predicting Later Cognitive Development

Does infant information processing, as measured in a habituation study, predict later cognitive functioning? When they first view a pattern or an object, infants will look at it ... sometimes for an extended period. However, if an infant sees the same pattern or object continuously or repeatedly, the infant (like you) develops a memory of it and eventually becomes bored, looking at the pattern or object less. That is, the infant has mentally processed information about the pattern or object. Infants differ in how quickly they process information in this way, and those individual differences appear to be meaningful. Bornstein and colleagues (2013) drew on a longitudinal study involving a large number of babies born in the United Kingdom. They measured habituation to a black-and-white checkerboard pattern when the infants were 4 months old. At 14 years, the adolescents completed standardized tests of English, mathematics, and science commonly used in British schools. Babies who habituated more efficiently at 4 months achieved higher academic scores at 14 years. Does this mean that an infant's intellectual abilities are set for life? The answer is "yes, but...". Yes, this kind of study indicates that infant information processing predicts adolescent cognition; however, the predictive relation is far from perfect, suggesting that other factors also affect children's eventual academic achievement. In addition, attentional skills (such as measured in habituation) are malleable. For example, people with ADHD are able to learn effective strategies to help offset attentional challenges.

Reaching the conclusion that infants can mentally represent the outside world opened an entirely new vista on thinking and the origins of thought, as well as the mental capabilities of babies. We now know that babies are capable of **representational thinking**, that is the ability to contemplate people and objects in their absence. Lev Vygotsky (1896–1934), a Russian psychologist, theorized that a critical development in infancy occurred with the advent of **interiorization**, the process of making the external world accessible to the internal mind (Vygotsky, 1934/1962). Piaget had ventured that a critical development in cognition occurred with the infant's achieving **object permanence**, knowing that an object was still there even though the infant could no longer see it. Of course, interiorization and object permanence are descriptions, not explanations. (*How* interiorization occurs is frankly a mystery which has not been solved to date, and we think summons to mind the parallel conundrum of consciousness, how organic tissue and electrochemical processes in the brain somehow give rise to awareness, thought, and all the wonderful dreams, desires, and feelings that make us human.) Along with representational thinking comes the ability to form and use **symbols** that anticipate memory, categorization, imitation, pretense, and language. Representational thinking is no small achievement.

Before the advent of representational thinking, young babies seem confused when it comes to symbolic relations. For example, younger infants appear to equate pictures with their real objects. Everyone who has read a picture book to a baby has seen the baby try to finger or grasp a picture as though it were a real object ... or even try to look behind the book to find the rest of the 3D object. A moment's reflection will reveal that the appreciation of picture books and screens calls on similar abilities. When and to what degree do infants think that what they see is actually real or only a representation? For these reasons, it is worth delving more deeply into the representational life of infants. To do so, we consider three topics that, in one way or another, illustrate the unveiling richness of mental representation in infancy. The three are categories and concepts, memory, and pretend play. Each reflects increasing mental sophistication and flexibility. Each also articulates with or is presumptive of language, which we cover formally in the next chapter.

CATEGORIES AND CONCEPTS

Categories are collections of things in the world, and concepts are the mental representation of those collections. Again, a bit of background will help to frame the high significance of categories and concepts to the mental life of infants. The world around us consists of an infinite number of properties and objects, events and people, and without conscious thought we group them into categories and represent them mentally as concepts. Categories collect together separate discriminable items into a set according to some rule. Members of a category may be grouped because they share a common attribute, element, or relation ("red things," "kitchen utensils," or "items that are human-made"), and the same property, object, event, or person can be categorized in different ways (at one level a dog is a member of the animal category, at another level a dog is a member of the living organism category). Categories have breadth (the variety of items included), boundaries (instances where inclusion is marginal), as well as prototypes (best examples). Consider the category of birds. Although all birds have feathers and beaks, birds vary in color, size, whether they fly, and preferred habitat. Thus, the bird category includes a wide variation. At the same time, categories have boundaries. Penguins do not fly, but they have other characteristics in common with birds, such as laying eggs. Prototypes are the best examples of a category possibly because they possess many (if not all) of the distinguishing features of the category, and when we think of a category, we often think in terms of prototypes. Robin, duck, and pigeon are prototypical birds; ostriches, penguins, and road runners are not.

Being able to categorize is enormously helpful to cognition. First, categorization structures and clarifies perception, helping to sort out James's blooming, buzzing confusion of infancy. The environment into which infants are born is complex and constantly changing, with many opportunities to encounter new properties and objects, events and people. Categorization helps to organize the environment. Categorization also facilitates learning. If infants have a category of animals, when seeing a new animal, they can rely on what they already know about animals and do not have to start anew to figure out all the properties of the new animal. Thus, infants can also use category knowledge to make inferences. For example, if shown a turtle and told it is an animal, an infant can infer that the turtle might eat, move, and breathe like other animals. Categorization also facilitates memory, especially the storage and retrieval of information. For example, all information pertaining to the animal category can be stored together and accessed when presented with familiar or novel animals.

Do infants categorize? Categorical perception of phonemes (discussed earlier) entailed infants treating distinguishable sounds ("ma"s) similarly. Infants to the same thing with color: Different shades of the same color are treated as the same. Infants also categorize across viewpoint, as illustrated in Figure 3.2. Another example is the categorization of the facial expression of smiling. Infants were habituated to four different intensities of smiles (Figure 3.7; Bornstein & Arterberry, 2003). Following habituation, infants looked significantly longer at a new and different facial expression (fear) than at a new and different intensity of smile, all on the same face, and when the expressions were modeled by different females. Categorization tells us that infants perceive the same expression across varying intensities or people modeling them. Turns out, infants categorize dimensions of their visual and auditory world all the time.

Categories are commonly structured by their "hierarchical inclusiveness" – more encompassing categories subsume less encompassing ones. For a simple example, a collie is a type of dog, which is a type of animal. At the highest level of category inclusiveness, often called the *superordinate* level (e.g., animal or vehicle in

Habituation

Test

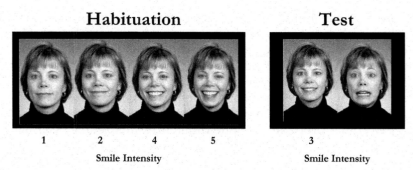

| 1 | 2 | 4 | 5 | | 3 |

Smile Intensity   Smile Intensity

Figure 3.7 Stimuli used to test 5-month-old infants' categorization of the facial expression of smiling. Note that in the test display the smile exemplar was not presented earlier in the habituation phase and that it represents a midpoint along the smile intensity continuum (1 is a slight smile and 5 is a broad toothy grin). (From Bornstein & Arterberry, 2003; reproduced with permission.)

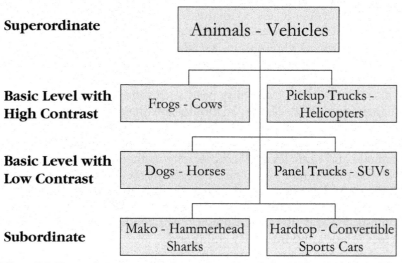

Superordinate — Animals - Vehicles

Basic Level with High Contrast — Frogs - Cows | Pickup Trucks - Helicopters

Basic Level with Low Contrast — Dogs - Horses | Panel Trucks - SUVs

Subordinate — Mako - Hammerhead Sharks | Hardtop - Convertible Sports Cars

Figure 3.8 Examples of superordinate, basic level, and subordinate categories. (Created by M. E. Arterberry, after Bornstein & Arterberry, 2010.)

Figure 3.8), category members are grouped functionally and share many perceptual attributes. For example, dogs, horses, rabbits, and fish all fall in the most inclusive category of animal because animals share many properties (they breathe, eat, and move on their own), but different animals do not (necessarily) look alike.

Moreover, the animal category differs from other high-level categories, such as vehicles, in instrumental and perceptual properties (e.g., both move but vehicles have motors and drivers and animals are self-propelled). At middle levels of inclusiveness, called the *basic level*, category members share instrumental and usually (although not always) perceptual properties. For example, dogs of different species share many characteristics as well as a number of perceptual properties despite differences in size (e.g., German Shepard versus Dachshund), and dogs are easily distinguished from fish. At the basic level members of a category can be highly distinctive or have high contrast, such as different colored frogs. At low levels of category inclusiveness, or the *subordinate level*, members of a category share both instrumental and perceptual similarity, however instrumental and perceptual similarity also tend to be high between categories. For example, mako sharks and hammerhead sharks are very similar in shape, function, and where they inhabit. Such hierarchical categorical systems are found widely across human cultures.

At what level or levels do infants first categorize? Developmental scientists make inferences about categorization based on patterns of infants' object exploration, as when infants sequentially touch or manipulate objects within a category (all the animals) more frequently than objects between categories (alternating between animals and vehicles). One study used such sequential touching with infants aged 12, 18, 24, and 30 months, testing each age group with seven object sets representing the levels depicted in Figure 3.8 (Bornstein & Arterberry, 2010). Infants at all ages categorized superordinate and basic level objects, as long as there was high contrast. Only 30-month-olds categorized objects at the basic level with low contrast, and no age group categorized at the subordinate level. Thus, the ability to notice, and perhaps care about, within-category similarities and between-category differences develops slowly across infancy and into early childhood.

Infants have many opportunities to learn about objects in their everyday experiences, and they use those experiences to guide their categorization. In one study, parents were given a picture book with totally novel objects to show their baby for 2 months, and they later brought the baby into the laboratory for a study of categorization of those objects. Infants' experiences with novel objects in the home facilitated their object categorization in the laboratory (Bornstein & Mash, 2010). A similar animal categorization advantage was shown by infants who have pets at home compared to those who do not (Kovack-Lesh et al., 2014).

MEMORY

It is obviously important that infants attend to properties, objects, events, and people in their environment and gain information about them, but it is also crucial that they be able to store, retrieve, and use that information. Elsewise, every moment would be new and novel to the infant. Look up from this book, close your eyes, and then open them. Now close them again and open them. Suppose every time you opened your eyes everything was new. How could thinking develop under such circumstances? Think too of the tragedy of Alzheimer's disease and what the loss of memory means. For years, scientists actually believed that infants could not remember much of anything because adults and even older children typically have few memories of anything that took place before the age of 3–4 years. Freud famously coined the term *infantile amnesia* to describe this phenomenon, which he attributed to the repression of memories of traumatic events. Piaget theorized that memory was not possible during the first year because it demands the capacity to think representationally, which he contended only emerged around 2 years of age. Developmental scientists have since learned that infants remember; indeed, babies hear *in utero* and after birth remember some of what they heard. We already saw one example: Newborns treat their mother's voice as familiar.

Memory is vital to our awareness, experience, knowledge, and interpretation of the world. Developmental scientists are interested in what infants can remember, in the nature of their memory representations, in the ways in which infants remember, and in how good infant memory is. A general rule is that memory develops across infancy as regions of the brain associated with memory (the hippocampus and thalamus) form and mature, and with age infants retain information for longer periods of time.

The habituation and novelty responsiveness procedures tap recognition memory (asking the question "have you seen this before?"). Both have proven to be versatile and powerful tools to investigate infant memory. Using habituation, it has been possible to track the rate at which infants encode stimulus material into memory. Presumably, faster habituation indexes quicker encoding. And, as pointed out in Chapter 1, by habituating infants and testing them immediately afterward with the same stimulus, it has been possible to study short-term recognition memory, just as imposing a delay between the end of habituation and a later test allows the study of long-term recognition memory. Similarly, comparing the rate of habituation to a stimulus at one time with the rate of habituation to the same stimulus at a later time, it has been possible to assess short- or long-term retention of the stimulus. If the second course of habituation is quicker than the first course, it must indicate that the infant remembered the stimulus.

Attention is a limiting factor in information processing and memory at all ages. To remember something, infants have to pay attention to it in the first place, and they have to know what aspects of a situation or event is worth attending to (Box 3.3). With age, infants increasingly focus on relevant aspects of to-be-remembered stimuli.

BOX 3.3   Screen Time for Baby?

There is a TV channel called *BabyTV* devoted exclusively to infant programming. Baby-targeted media typically combine visual and auditory stimuli (e.g., 3D objects floating in space along with music), and some have words (spoken, written, and sometimes signed with American Sign Language) paired with objects. With most parents owning a smart phone or tablet, infants experience an estimated 53 minutes of screen media per day.

Infants' exposure to screen media raises a number of questions (Myers & Arterberry, 2022), but the one germane to this chapter on thinking is whether babies understand and remember the information presented in videos. Certainly, videos are attention-getting. For example, 12- to 18-month-olds attend to 65% of a *Baby Mozart* video (Barr et al., 2008), and parents believe that their children learn from videos (Rideout & Hamel, 2006). But do babies actually learn and remember?

DeLoache and her colleagues (2010) addressed this question. They asked one group of parents to show their 12- to 18-month-olds a popular DVD several times a week for 4 weeks. The DVD had a variety of scenes of a house and a yard and a voice labeled common objects. Half of the parents (Group 1) were asked to also interact with their infants while watching the DVD, and the other half (Group 2) were asked to allow their infants to watch the DVD without interacting with their children. Two more groups of parents and infants who did not watch the video also participated in this study. Group 3 parents were asked to try to teach their children a list of 25 words (the same words presented in the DVD), and Group 4 was a control condition in which only the infants' vocabulary was assessed. After 4 weeks, all infants were tested for their vocabulary knowledge. Children in Group 3 learned the most words when their parents tried to teach them the words, and children in Groups 1 and 2 (the DVD conditions with and without interaction) learned the fewest words. Notably, the performance by the DVD infants was not different from the control Group 4.

One barrier to learning is making the connection between the object on the screen and real objects. Thus, exposing infants to baby-targeted media does not appear to facilitate learning. Consistent with other research on this video deficit (Anderson & Pempek, 2005; Strouse & Samson, 2021), it appears that direct interaction with people and objects is the best context for promoting infants' learning about and remembering the world around them.

Context is important to memory. Context refers to features of the internal and external environments that are present during information processing. Recall the mobile kicking method of learning described in Chapter 1. In one study, 3-month-olds learned in the foot-kicking paradigm while they were surrounded by colorful crib bumpers. Changes in the bumper did not affect their retention of the contingency 1 day later when the memory was fresh. However, after delays of 3, 5, and 7 days, infants successfully remembered the contingency only when the bumpers surrounding the crib during the retention test matched the bumpers present during training (Rovee-Collier & Cuevas, 2009). Parents sometimes report being surprised by what their babies remember. We were surprised too when we tested babies at 5 months in an uncomfortable social interaction with a female they had never seen before (called the still-face paradigm described in Chapter 4; Bornstein et al., 2004). A full 14 months later, the infants viewed videos of that woman and two other appearance-matched females. These infants avoided looking at the woman they saw at 5 months, suggesting that they remembered something about that uncomfortable interaction for over 1 year!

PLAY

It might seem odd to include play in a discussion of infant thinking and mental representation. Isn't play social? Of course, it is. Play is certainly fun and interactive. But play also involves looking at a stuffed animal, manipulating a busy box, building with a set of blocks, and entertaining at a make-believe tea party. Play also frequently imitates life, and it is common to find older infants re-enacting specific events that they observe or participate in routinely ("driving" a toy car). The advent of pretend play (as well as language) during the second year of life reflects an underlying developmental progression in infants' capacities to represent events mentally.

Play is a perfect stage on which infants exhibit physical, motor, mental, linguistic, and socioemotional competencies. In bold outline, play begins as simple inspection and manipulation and moves gradually to sophisticated pretense and symbolism. In many ways, play is an important type of self-initiated infant learning.

Piaget was among the first developmental scientists to study infant play seriously because he saw infant play as a platform for integrating different mental abilities and as support for his theory that mental development depends on motor activity and interactions in the world. Play is exploration, and how exploration unfolds reveals much about mental development. Piaget learned about play again from closely watching his own three young children, but the lessons he learned have withstood the test of time and appear to apply generally to infancy.

1.   Action is the basis of knowledge. Younger infants first manipulate one object at a time with one action at a time (mouthing, pushing, pulling). Next, older infants manipulate the parts of objects or several objects together as if studying relations among them (putting a spoon into a cup). Then, infants play with an object in the way the object was intended to be played with (rolling a toy car on its wheels across the floor). After, infants bring together unrelated objects (a spoon and a block) with no indication of pretense until they bring together two objects in a meaningful and appropriate way (stirring a spoon inside a cup). At these stages, play appears designed to extract information about objects, what objects do, what perceivable qualities they have, and what immediate effects they can produce.

2.   Infant play development is sequential, moving from concrete and nonsymbolic actions to representational pretense and symbolic actions, or the use of one object to stand for another or pretending to engage in an action (such as putting a banana to sleep at bedtime).

3.   Pretend play shifts from play involving only the self (pretending to sleep) through pretend play involving self–object relations (pretending to drink from a cup) to pretend play involving objects exclusively (having a doll pretend to drink).

Infant play supports thinking and learning. During and as the result of play, infants acquire information and skills, engage in creative and divergent thinking, and attain more sophisticated representational abilities.

These very general lessons apply across infants. Of course, as with all other capacities, play is hallmarked by individual differences in the rates at which individual infants achieve representation and their levels of achievement. For example, in one study 15% of 13-month-olds' total play was symbolic, but some individual 13-month-olds never exhibited symbolic play, whereas as much as 51% of the play of others was symbolic (Tamis-LeMonda & Bornstein, 1990). At 20 months, 31% of infants' total play was symbolic, but some individual 20-month-olds showed as little as 2% symbolic play, whereas for others 83% of play was symbolic. Furthermore, infants who showed more representational play at 13 months also showed more representational play at 20 months – but this stability depended on the involvement of infants' mothers.

Many early researchers looked at play as a solitary child activity. In contrast, Vygotsky proposed that social interaction fosters the growth of symbolic functioning in children, and he used play as a prime example. The infant's achievement of symbolic play is now seen as a reflection of the infant's individual growth in the context of interpersonal interactions and sociocultural setting (you guessed it, the transaction of nature and nurture). Play emerges in infants, but adults influence its development by outfitting their infants' play environment, engaging infants actively, and responding to infants' play overtures. That is, mothers who know more about play tend to prompt their children to play at more sophisticated levels than do mothers with less accurate knowledge.

Importantly, were we to observe infants playing by themselves with a set of toys and record the kinds of play they engage in, we would see infants of a given age playing at some of the levels Piaget described. If, however, we were then to observe the same infants with the same toys play with their mothers, we would see the same infants playing at higher Piagetian levels. That is, the play of 20-month-olds with their mothers is more sophisticated, complex, and varied than the same infants' play when alone. What mothers do with their infants during play affects the quality of their infants' play. Mothers of 20-month-olds who initiate symbolic play more frequently have infants who engage in symbolic play more frequently. Mothers and infants appear to be attuned to each other during play, with the play level of one partner being closely geared to the play level of the other. We return to these mutual mother-infant relations in Chapter 6 on Relating.

SUMMARY

The start of this chapter posed the question of whether infants think. Here at the end we can conclude that infants enjoy a surprisingly rich mental life – infants sense, perceive, learn, process information, remember, categorize, and play. Their representational abilities attest that infants enjoy multiple capacities to acquire, share, and use information about the environment. Indeed, from the very beginning of life babies actively seek out information, and rapidly thereafter their perceptual world becomes organized. Babies distinguish and attend to properties of objects as well as to relations among properties. Infants categorize perceptual qualities and objects. They imitate others, and they remember properties, objects, events, and people. And finally, they learn and grow cognitively through play. Neither nativist nor empiricist theorists own an understanding of infant mental development; rather, infant and experience co-construct infant cognition. Endogenous (internal, biological) and exogenous (external, experiential) forces work together to bring the infant's mind in line with the physical and social realities in the world.

COMMUNICATING

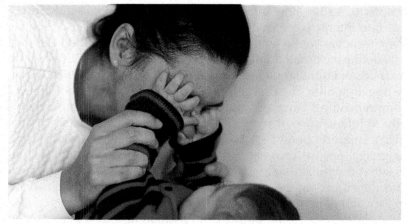

(Image courtesy of Shutterstock, copyright: True Touch Lifestyle/ Shutterstock.com.)

INTRODUCTION

During just 1 year of postnatal life, infants pass many milestones as the first chapters in this book relate. Their nervous systems mature rapidly, and their bodies grow at an equally impressive rate. In addition, they quickly come to sense and perceive the world around them in sophisticated ways, and they think – they learn, process information, imitate, mentally represent, categorize, remember, and

DOI: 10.4324/9781003172802-4

play. By the second half of the first year, many infants also know life routines that repeat every day: Getting ready to eat, take a bath, and go to sleep. While crawling, they know where they want to go, and by raising their arms they clearly indicate they want to be carried. Next to the speed of nervous system, physical, sensory, perceptual, and mental development, actually speaking oddly lags far behind.

Every parent has sensed their baby feeling, wanting, and knowing but at the same time flummoxed in being unable simply to express those feelings, wants, and thoughts. Infants commonly resort to crying, tugging, and grunting to communicate. The nonverbal state of affairs can be deeply frustrating for both parent and child, which makes infants' first words – when they finally arrive – all the more cause for celebration.

In the estimation of many parents (never mind developmental scientists), children only leave infancy when they begin to communicate verbally with those around them. However, "conversations" with babies begin well before words come into consideration. This chapter describes how infants develop from speechless individualists into interactive conversationalists, ready and able to articulate their feelings, wants, and thoughts to others. To set the stage, we first define the broad domains of language. Next, we briefly describe methods of infant language study. The bulk of the chapter settles on two main topics. The first concerns the beginning stages of infants' comprehending language and their vocalizations leading eventually to infants' use of words. The second main topic concerns the many supports parents provide infants on their way to acquiring language. Special characteristics of speech to children and activities that teach turn-taking facilitate infants' language development and their learning the social uses of language. Despite their seeming incompetence, infants are surprisingly prepared and remarkably plastic, possessing both the motivation and the competencies to ensure that they will become full participants in language. The chapter concludes with a discussion of multilingualism, remarking on its ascendancy and importance for understanding the real world of infant language development. Faithful to the whole-child view, language coalesces impressive accomplishments in the nervous, physical, perceptual, cognitive, and social spheres of development.

DOMAINS OF LANGUAGE

For all the ease and automaticity adults show in speaking and understanding, human language is an extremely complicated business. To go forward with explicating its origins in infancy, we need a bit of

	Phonology	Semantics	Syntax	Pragmatics
Comprehension				
Production				

Figure 4.1 The language domain matrix for acquiring one language. (Created by M. H. Bornstein.)

background. Language involves several broad domains. **Phonology** is concerned with sounds that are used in language. **Semantics** (vocabulary or lexicon) involve words and their meaning. **Syntax** (grammar) defines the ways in which words and phrases are combined, structured, and meaningfully arranged. **Pragmatics** entails social rules that dictate everyday language usage (e.g., using *please* and *thank you*, taking turns in conversation). All four domains also have two faces. One is comprehension, that is understanding sounds, vocabulary, grammar, and social rules. The other is production, that is saying the sounds and vocabulary and using grammar and social rules. So minimally, acquiring language entails mastering all the cells of a 2 × 4 table (Figure 4.1).

Consider all that infants must do simply to understand what their parents mean when they say, *OhJuju!Wheredidthedoggiego?* The infant must segregate the sounds in the speech stream into individual words, map meaning onto each word, and analyze the grammatical structure that links the words. For example, how do babies know that *Juju*, *here*, and *doggie* are different words as opposed to *ohju*, *thed*, and *giego*, that *Juju* is a name (for the child or the dog), let alone what *go* means (run versus disappear versus urinate), or that *doggie* is an animal? All this decoding must take place in real time as that complex utterance unfolds. Anyone who is not a proficient speaker of a second language traveling in the country of that language will readily empathize with the infants' plight. Young infants with mental capacities far less advanced than adults nonetheless rapidly become quite good first understanding and later speaking, despite the abstractness and complexity of language.

Infants first need to learn how their language sounds and what sounds are likely to go together. By hearing your language, say English, you know that "*hj*" cannot start a word, and this gives you a head start in decoding because you can rule out "*O hjuju ...*". Of course, this is not a complete solution – there is nothing un-English about a possible word like "*thed*" – but it is a start. Each language has many other such helpful regularities. By 2 to 6 months, infants prefer to listen to speech more than complex nonspeech sounds, and by the middle of the first year infants prefer to listen to sounds consistent with those of their own language. This kind of knowledge is really helpful for meeting the challenge of discovering which elements of the continuous speech stream are words.

Like other areas of infant development, questions about the roles of nature and nurture in infants' acquisition of language are long-standing. Arguing for nature, the Emperor Constantine (272–337) opined that language emerges with the natural eruption of infants' baby teeth, and the U.S. linguist Noam Chomsky (1928–) proposed that language acquisition depends on inborn predispositions. Arguing for nurture, St. Augustine (354–430) wrote that children learn language by imitation, and Skinner asserted that children learn language operantly through reinforcement of their vocalizations. We think that language is too rich, unique, and complex a system for infants simply to learn, just as it is too rich, unique, and complex a system for newborns simply to know. As we have seen with earlier topics and as this chapter argues, language development has biological roots at the same time that it depends on experience.

BACK TO NORMS AND INDIVIDUAL DIFFERENCES

Next, consider the general course of language acquisition. Figure 4.2 shows in a simplified way some milestones of language development in infancy. Three principles are noteworthy in this display. First, comprehension precedes production. Just like adults understand many more words than they use every day, infants understand more language than they speak. Infants respond to speaking voices long before they say their first simple syllables. Infants are thought to first understand words at around 9 months but not say any words until around 12 months or later on average; children reach another milestone of understanding 50 words at around 12 months, but they do not produce 50 words until around 18 months or later. The fact that infants generally understand more than they can say means that language develops covertly. In other words, infants' language progress is not clearly reflected in what they say. The regularity of these comprehension-production differences, as well as the existence of general norms, seem to support a strong role for biology in language acquisition.

The second clear principle from Figure 4.2 is the notable degree of variation. Each language achievement has a bandwidth indicating the range of individual differences. At 13 months, some infants

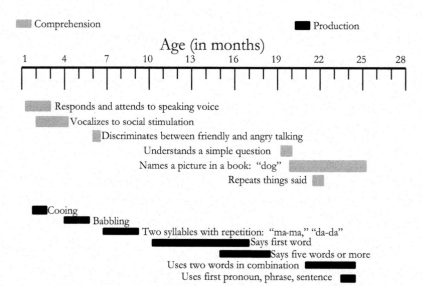

Figure 4.2 Approximate age norms for the development of comprehension and production of language in infants over the first 2½ years of life. (Created by M. E. Arterberry.)

comprehend 10 words, others 75; some produce 0 words, others almost 30. At 20 months, individual children have productive vocabularies ranging from 8 to 434 words! This incredible range of individual variation is true of children learning most all languages. One study of seven languages recorded that 20-month-olds range from as few as 1 spoken word to as many as 487 (Bornstein et al., 2004). A practical example is when babies can be expected to recognize their own name. Most developmental psycholinguists estimate that infants will respond to their first name sometime between 4 and 10 months, but infants saying their name (or the names of others) might not emerge until 18 to 24 months. So, here again the watchword is individual differences. Of course, a one-syllable name like *Paul* is short and so might appear early; Elon Musk and singer Claire Boucher (better known by her stage name, Grimes) named their son *X Æ A-12 Musk*, so when he first recognized or said his name is anyone's guess. These pervasive individual differences support both nature (likely some variation reflects differential brain maturation in different children) as well as nurture (likely some variation reflects the different experiences with language different children enjoy). Importantly, quantitative individual differences in language acquisition are complemented by qualitative differences (Box 4.1).

BOX 4.1   Qualitative Differences in Infant Language

Beside quantitative differences among infants in language development, infants fall into different styles of language production. So-called **referential** children have high proportions of nouns in their vocabularies, whereas so-called **expressive** children use more pronouns and action words, and their speech is populated with social formulae and routines. One developmental scientist described these two children on the basis of videorecording them at play with their mothers at home at 12, 15, and 18 months (Goldfield, 1985/1986):

- *Johanna* is a referential child. Of Johanna's first 50 words, 49 were names for things (e.g., keys, nose). In play, approximately one-half of her attempts to engage her mother involved her giving or showing a toy (ball), and reciprocally Johanna's mother consistently labeled toys for her ("It's a ball.").
- *Caitlin* is an expressive child. Only 35% of Caitlin's first words consisted of names for things. Instead, her early lexicon consisted of social expressions, many of them in phrases (e.g., "Thank you", "Hey guys!"). She included a toy in fewer than one-fifth of her bids to her mother, preferring instead to engage in routines of social play (peek-a-boo).

These two styles of communicating appear to function differently for children. For referential children, the purpose of language is to label, describe, and exchange information; whereas, for expressive children, language denotes or confirms social interaction. Of course, Caitlin and Johanna are extremes. Most language-learning infants exhibit a more balanced picture of referential and expressive speech. In fact, a given child may sometimes look referential and other times expressive, depending on the context or demands of a situation.

Not shown in Figure 4.2 are several implications from this second principle of variation. One is that infants who comprehend more words are also likely to produce more words. Another is that these individual differences are relatively long-lasting. Infants who understand and say more words early in life become children with larger speaking and reading vocabularies. Developmental scientists who study the growth of language in this way have referred to this phenomenon as the "Matthew effect" (after the passage in the Bible, Matthew 25:29, where it is basically written that *the rich get richer and the poor get poorer*). Others call it the language gap, one that widens as children age.

The third principle from Figure 4.2 is increasing complexity. Both comprehension and production get more complex and sophisticated by the month. In the first month, infants respond to the human voice; by 24 months, toddlers comprehend the meaning of prepositions ("Lewis, put the ball in the basket."). Infants babble at around 6 to 8 months of age, and enter the two-word stage at around 24 months. Vocabulary is thought to "spurt" as soon as infants realize that things have names. This epiphany is called **nominal insight,** and having achieved it infants suddenly begin labeling objects and learning new words rapidly.

HOW DO WE KNOW WHAT CHILDREN UNDERSTAND AND SAY?

Our picture of infants' developing language rests on parent report, observation, and testing. A lot of the early work in child language focused on production and was done by parents, many of whom were themselves linguists and who kept diaries of their own infant's first language. This approach involved intensive analyses of infants' spontaneous speech. Related is a more generic strategy that employs parents as reporters where parents (usually mothers) are interviewed or now more usually complete checklists of words that their infant understands or says. Objective knowledge of infants' language comes from observation - listening to infants, recording them, and analyzing transcripts of child speech. Testing includes scales where infants demonstrate their comprehension of increasingly difficult verbal expressions by pointing to named objects or enacting a phrase (such as putting the ball in the basket) or elicited production tasks that ask children to name objects or produce verbs such as *today she is walking; yesterday she " ___ "*. Notably, these different measures of infant language tend to agree with one another. Parents who report that their infants know and speak in more sophisticated ways have infants who by independent observation use more words and longer utterances in everyday speech with their parents. Also, the same infants comprehend and produce more words when tested by experimenters.

At the same time, for reasons reviewed in Chapter 1, there are advantages and disadvantages to each method – report, observation, and test. Children's verbal abilities can differ depending on the social and physical contexts in which they are measured. Infants are chatty in the bath, but nearly every infant has failed to say something for a grandparent that the same infant (even minutes before!) repeatedly said to the parents. Free play elicits some linguistic skills from infants, whereas language while eating can be expected to be quite different. The most reliable information about child language comes when several measurement techniques are used together.

COMPREHENDING LANGUAGE

Language competency requires that infants achieve in two dimensions: They need to understand meaning in others' speech – in short, comprehend language – and they must encode meaning into their own speech so that others can understand them – in short, produce language. These twin competencies are not in synch, as language comprehension typically precedes language production; that is, well before they speak infants give every indication that they understand a good amount of language. By 6 months infants are thought to recognize that *Mommy* names the child's caregiver, and by 8 months infants are thought to be sensitive to grammatical patterns in their native language. Like perception, however, infants' language comprehension is private, and parents and developmental scientists alike must infer that infants comprehend on the basis of their behaviors, not their speech. In consequence, there is a large guessing element to understand infant language comprehension. Yet, we do know that by the second year of life, comprehension has run so far ahead of production that it is really difficult to know how many words, for example, a given infant really understands.

PRODUCING LANGUAGE

Infants take three big steps in starting to speak: The first is prelinguistic, the second is using one word, and the third is using many words to create phrases or sentences. Two early types of prelinguistic vocalizations are crying and babbling. An infant's cry is very revealing about normal and atypical development because cries are both communicative and diagnostic. Different infant physiological states, such as hunger and sleepiness, are associated with different patterns of crying, and female adults (especially mothers) show special and different brain responses to cries versus other emotional sounds. Most adults can neither deny nor disregard a baby's cry: Infants' cries compel us to respond, and the nearly universal response is to be nurturing in some way. Cries are also diagnostic of problems in development, as infants with various medical conditions (such as prematurity or autism) make different distress cry sounds from typically developing infants, and they cry more than typically developing infants.

BABBLING

Pre-speech non distress vocalizations consist of many different simple sounds and may be vegetative, like sneezing and burping, or vocalic, like cooing and trilling. Their squeals, growls, and yells demonstrate infants' seeming playful exploration of their own vocal tract capabilities. Infant's first babbles appear about the middle of the first year. Babbling is composed of repetitive consonant-vowel sequences of syllables (like "*da-da-da*") and sequences of different consonants and vowels (like "*ba-ga-da*"). Babbling sounds like fun, and it fills the eerie void between silence and crying so common in early infancy. But, babbling also is the first significant type of non distress communication. Babbling appears to be wired into infants' brains (or hands, as is the case for deaf babies who manually babble). Babbling gives evidence of both biological and experiential influences: Spanish-, Japanese-, and English-learning babies show no great differences in their babbling sound production repertoires, however babbling has the tonal qualities of the target language babies will eventually speak.

If all of this sounds easy, it is not. Developmental psycholinguists have accurately labeled speech production among the most complex of human action patterns. Speaking requires the brain's exquisite coordination of movements of the mouth, tongue, and lips with the outflow of air from the lungs. Sound production is constrained by the anatomy of the vocal tract and mouth (Emperor Constantine was on to something regarding the role of teeth), and anatomical constraints in the infant underpin an interesting developmental story regarding parenting and infancy. The Russian linguist Roman Jakobson (1896–1982) proposed the romantic view that infants' first vocalizations reflect a restricted set of sound contrasts that follow a universal pattern related to roles that the mouth and vocal tract play in uttering sounds. Some consonant sounds are produced primarily at the lips in the front of the mouth (*m* and *p* are examples), others by positioning the tongue against the teeth (*d* is an example), and others at the back of the mouth (*g* is an example). Vowel sounds (*o, e*, and *a*) are articulated at roughly parallel points from the front to the back of the mouth. Jakobson proposed that articulation of consonants follows a general developmental progression from front to back and that of vowels from back to front. This means that infants' earliest vocal combinations ought to be front consonants with back vowels: that is, *m* or *p* or *d* with *a*. Close listening reveals that infants produce syllables sounding like *ma* and *pa* relatively more often than, say, *eg*. It also does not escape notice that the sound combinations with the highest probability of appearing first in infant vocalizations, based on Jakobson's theory, tend to be those that connote important people in early life, ma, pa, and da. A survey of 1,072 languages showed that almost 60% use *ma*-like, *pa*-like, and *da*-like sounds as parental kin terms. The implication seems to be that parents (or languages) have directly adopted generic labels for themselves based on infants' earliest, anatomically determined vocal productions (and also why *Paul* might also be easier to say than *X Æ A-12*).

Infants' early speech production is more sophisticated than it sounds to our naked ears. When infants first start saying words, they seem to fail to make certain distinctions clear. An infant might be heard to pronounce *pa* and *ba* at the beginnings of different words exactly the same. However, technical analyses of vocal recordings of infants have revealed that infants actually enunciate the sounds differently, but not differently enough for adults to hear the distinction (Macken & Barton, 1980). This kind of technologically aided finding echoes a theme that has arisen again and again in the study of language development. The roots of complex behaviors may be discovered long before those behaviors are clear and overt, and many infant capacities that seem to bloom overnight have in fact been emerging in more rudimentary forms for months. Developmental scientists recognize this continuity between infants' babbling and their early words. Both rest on the same articulatory mechanisms, they share many of the same fundamental speech sounds, and first words often incorporate frequently produced babbling sounds.

WORDS

Infants cry, babble, and gesture to communicate effectively long before they actually use words. But these pre-linguistic methods of communication are hampered by severe limitations. It is impossible for an infant to use gestures to share a memory, and all parents attest to their frustrations at decoding the inherent ambiguity of infant cries and babbles. The next big step is for infants to learn that sounds connect to meanings and that specific sounds connect to specific meanings in their specific language. Infants are non speakers, and so strictly speaking speech per se is not a part of this book, but we would be remiss to abandon the reader of a book on infancy at the doorstep of such a momentous advance.

Perhaps the major obstacle confronting the language-learning infant is the problem of **reference**, linking a sound with a meaning. Recall once again *OhJuju!Wheredidthedoggiego?* This time consider that, to understand this simple statement, even after parsing the speech stream into separate units correctly, the infant (*"Juju"*) must determine which spoken unit refers to the infant, which to objects (*"doggie,"*) in the environment, which to an action (*"go"*), and so forth. After all, connections between word sounds and word meanings are essentially arbitrary. Any sound could go with any meaning After all, different languages work by having different sounding names for the same thing. This situation makes the infant's decoding task especially challenging.

Some language achievements challenge comprehension or production. Reference is a challenge to both. Even the most basic aspect of defining what an infant's first word is is a challenge. Is *baba* (for bottle) a real word even if the infant uses *baba* consistently to refer to a bottle and nothing else but a bottle? Some developmental scientists argue yes ... sounds label objects. Others say no ... *baba* is not a word in English (for example), and the infant has to say the word *bottle* for it to count as a word. Still others contend that even *bottle* cannot be counted as a word until it is applied to any bottle and not just the infant's specific bottle.

A related challenge to crediting infants with word knowledge turns on a usage distinction. Many infants use single sounds in regular or stereotyped ways, such as saying *baba* consistently to refer to a bottle. Infants might not have mastered pronunciations and word meanings that are aligned with those in their language, but such an accomplishment indicates that they have taken the important step of using certain sounds regularly to mean certain things, even if their use only occurs in a specific and limited way. Regardless of the argument over what a word is, developmental psycholinguists agree that understanding that things have names (nominal insight) is a big deal. However, there are more and less conservative construals of nominal insight. A less conservative construal – context-restricted – is where an infant might say *baba* to refer only to the infant's own bottle. Some authorities contend that using words in this way does not evidence true nominal insight because the word (*baba*) is not applied to a class (in this case, all bottles). More conservative authorities do not credit infants with nominal insight until infants use words like *baba* in a more general - context-flexible - way, that is even when the referent (bottle) is not present (see Box 4.2)

BOX 4.2   The Problem of Word Learning

Word learning is an example of a form of reasoning called **induction**, using a limited set of examples to draw conclusions that permit inferences about new cases: *I've seen that living things like cats, dogs, and my sister all breathe, so a living giraffe I've never seen before also likely breathes.* Suppose an infant sees a cup and simultaneously hears the word *cup*. For the infant to recognize that the same word also refers to other cups requires induction: going beyond the taught example to other instances.

Achieving induction is not as simple as it sounds. Put yourself for a moment in infants' shoes and consider two immediate problems. First, there is the *reference problem*: What do speakers mean when they say *cup*? Sometimes speakers will be pointing to an object when labeling it, but even in these seemingly clear cases the word *cup* might refer to many possible things. It might mean the cup, but it could also mean the handle, hot liquid, drinking, not appropriate for babies your age, or any of an infinite number of other conceivable meanings. Second, there is the *extension problem*. Once infants have guessed which particular entity is referred to, they should then be willing to extend this word to other entities belonging to the same category (unless the word is a proper name). But what makes a cup a cup? Its shape? color? function? We cannot simply say, "things that are similar to the original cup" because without a definition of similarity, we are right back where we started. How do infants get it right?

Developmental psycholinguists have identified three so-called **constraints** that infants might use when learning words. One is the **whole object constraint**. Under this argument, it is assumed that, when adults point to an object and label it, infants first perceive that the novel label refers to the whole object, and not to its parts, substance, or other properties. The cup is the cup and not the handle, etc. Second is the **taxonomic constraint**. Under this argument, it is assumed that infants interpret new words as referring to the object that they first see labeled with a word and interpret nouns as category labels for other objects that are the same kind of thing and not to properties. In one experiment, infants heard a novel label (*This is a blicket*) for a novel object (a purple horse). Then they were shown a contrasting object, an orange carrot, and they heard *this is not a blicket*. Finally, infants viewed two objects, a green horse and a purple chair, and were asked to *find the blicket*. Infants as young as 14 months looked to the green horse, extending the word *blicket* to the object category (horses) but not to a color (purple) (Booth & Waxman, 2009). Third is the **exclusivity constraint**. Under this argument, any given object has only one name (at least for children learning only one language). Thus, it is assumed that new words typically refer to unfamiliar objects, rather than objects that already have a known label.

Word learning constraints describe infants' behavior but do not explain it. Word learning is also not limited to object labels. After all, many of infants' first words are not names for things. Verbs refer to visible actions (*jumping*) and to non observable processes (*thinking*). Infants need to match verbs with actions, some of which are visible and some of which are not. Thus, there is still a lot to learn about how infants amass large vocabularies in such a short period of time.

As a rough rule of thumb, infants utter their first words around their first birthday (coincidentally when their first teeth erupt). What do infants' first words usually refer to? Two simple predictions might be that (1) infants' first words are those that they hear most often and that (2) the part of speech (noun, verb, adjective, etc.) of infants' first words would be proportional to the number of words infants hear of each part. Surprisingly, Prediction 1 turns out not to be supported. The two most frequent words in English-language speech to infants are "*you*" and "*the*," which rarely, if ever, make even the top 50 words infants first produce. Prediction 2 is supported by research, but not for the reason given. Most studies of English (and other languages) have found that the largest number of infants' early words are nouns; however, nouns do not necessarily occupy this pride of place because infants hear more nouns than other parts of speech. Recordings testify that mothers speaking Western languages (such as English and German) say more nouns than verbs, but mothers speaking in Eastern languages (such as Japanese, Korean, and Chinese) say more verbs than nouns. Infants learning both Western and Eastern languages still have more nouns than verbs in their early vocabularies. Why?

Developmental scientists have offered three main explanations for the early noun advantage but settled on none. One possibility is that nouns often refer to concrete objects which infants can see and feel, whereas verbs refer to visible actions (*jump*) but also invisible actions (*think*) and relations (*are*). Notions like *dog* are therefore easier to grasp than notions like *give*. A second possibility is that nouns are learned more readily because it is easier for infants to identify which aspects of a scene adults are talking about when they use nouns than when they use verbs. It is not the concepts themselves that are hard to grasp, but it is identifying which concept adults are using a word for. A third possibility is that many nouns tend to be used the same way – to refer to things – so once you learn a few nouns, learning more nouns is easy because they refer to similar kinds of categories. By contrast, verbs are more heterogeneous, referring to movements (*go*), desires (*want, like*), manipulations of objects (*put, get*), and so forth, and infants need to understand the concepts behind the words before understanding the verb referring to them.

Once infants attain about 50 words in their vocabulary, word learning appears to proceed rapidly. If lexical size estimates are at all accurate, the average 3-year-old possesses a vocabulary of 3,000 words. Therefore, between approximately 12 and 36 months, children acquire four new words per day on average. The average

6-year-old might command 14,000 words (Templin, 1957). In reaching these achievements, children demonstrate not only perceptual attentiveness, but mental absorptiveness: Babies are keen and adventurous language sponges.

SUPPORTS FOR INFANT LANGUAGE LEARNING

Infants bring a developing brain (Box 4.3) plus their winning personalities to acquire quickly the complex, dynamic, and symbolic system that is language. In accomplishing this challenging task, infants are not ill-equipped, nor are they alone. Chapter 6 on Relating examines some of the many ways that caregiver-infant interactions propel infant development generally. But caregivers directly affect children's acquisition of language, and from quite early in life. A laboratory experiment demonstrates that babies' vocalizations can be operantly conditioned through contingent social reinforcement. In this study, one group of mothers was instructed to respond

---

BOX 4.3   Sources of Language Development: Nature and Nurture Again

Nature. Human language depends on a human brain; every non human species possesses a brain, but no non human species has language like humans have. Certain structures in the human brain are involved in particular aspects of language processing: *Broca's area* (in the left frontal lobe) is associated with producing language, and *Wernicke's area* (in the left temporal lobe) is associated with comprehending language (we know this because insults to these specific areas, like injury or strokes, affect those specific aspects of language processing). Listening to words activates left frontotemporal areas about 400 milliseconds (4 tenths of a second) after their onset in 12- to 18-month-olds similar to what is found in adult word comprehension tasks (Travis et al., 2011). Specialization of the left temporal areas for language processing likely starts earlier than 1 year of age and may be present as soon as 1 month. Moreover, infants with larger productive vocabularies show stronger ERPs in left temporal areas than infants with smaller vocabularies (Friedrich & Friederici, 2010). Thus, the growing infant brain prepares the infant for language.

Furthermore, the drive to communicate appears to be innate, and putting words together in meaningful ways is thought to be wired into infants' nature. A group of parents of deaf infants of normal intelligence prohibited their babies from learning manual sign language (Goldin-Meadow, 2006). As a consequence, these infants had essentially no experience with any formal language (spoken or signed), although their other life experiences were normal. These children eventually made up their own gestural language. When the communicative gestures of these infants were recorded and categorized into individual units (analogous to words) and connected multi-sign units (analogous to phrases), it emerged that these deaf infants had developed signs to refer to objects, people, and actions, and they combined signs into ordered phrases to express relations among words. Moreover, the timing of the infants' invention of communication systems roughly paralleled that of hearing-normal infants learning spoken languages – their first "words" appeared at around 12 months, and their first combinations of words appeared several months later.

Nurture. All children use two sources of information when beginning to speak: the speech they hear and feedback from their own speech. This chapter delves more deeply into the many experiential supports afforded infants for language learning. For example, variation in the vocabularies of language-learning infants can be traced to environmental factors such as the type and amount of parent speech, and deaf infants who cannot hear their own speech almost never learn to speak with normal enunciation (although, of course, their language production in sign may be perfectly fluent). Thus, auditory input experience is necessary for the normal and timely development of language.

Nature *and* Nurture. Of course, infants need a maturing brain to process language, but experience with language doubtlessly shapes the course of brain development. We use our brains to understand and speak our language, but what language our brains understand and speak depends on the language we experienced as infants.

contingently whenever their infants' babbled, that is to give social feedback by smiling, moving closer to the infant, and/or touching their child. A second group of otherwise similar mothers was instructed to respond whenever the experimenter told them to, and experimenters arranged it so that mothers' actions were not contingent on their infants' babbling. Infants who received contingent responses increased in their number of speech sounds, and they even restructured their babbling to incorporate patterns from their mothers' speech (Goldstein & Schwade, 2008). Contingent responsiveness is but one example of the everyday activities that caregivers engage in to help infants acquire language. Others include infant-directed speech, labeling, joint attention, gaze following, and pointing and gesturing. Also, parents facilitate infants learning to take turns, a central component of true conversation.

INFANT-DIRECTED SPEECH

Unwittingly, parents repackage language aimed at infants to match infant capacities. Mothers, fathers, caregivers, and even adults who are not parents regularly adopt a special dialect when addressing infants: We have previously referred to it, and it is variously called *baby talk, motherese, parentese,* or more neutrally **infant-directed speech**. Infant-directed speech includes special characteristics and modifications of adult-directed speech in practically all domains of language. At the sound level, infant-directed speech uses higher pitch (fundamental frequency), a greater range of frequencies, and more varied and exaggerated intonations. Simplicity features include using shorter utterances, a slower tempo, longer pauses between phrases, fewer embedded clauses, and fewer auxiliary verbs. Redundancy features more repetition over shorter amounts of time and more immediate repetitions. Lexical features include special forms (like *mama*). Content features include a restriction of topics to the infants' world. Infant-directed speech is similar to the way people speak to their pets, and it simulates a general form of communication used between lovers (who are known to call one another *baby*).

Infant-directed speech appears to be intuitive, non conscious, and widespread. Bilingual mothers use it in both languages they speak to their infants, and deaf mothers modify their sign language in the same ways hearing mothers use infant-directed speech. Children as young as 4 years of age even engage in many of the same systematic language adjustments when speaking to an infant. Cross-cultural research also confirms that infant-directed speech is essentially universal. A frequently investigated feature of infant-directed speech is the alteration of pitch. Analyses of recordings of the fundamental frequencies of mothers and fathers speaking French, Italian, German, Japanese, British English, and American English to their preverbal infants (as opposed to another adult) revealed a cross-language consistency in this speech modification. Mothers and fathers alike used higher mean, minimum, and maximum pitch and a greater variability in pitch. They also used shorter utterances and longer pauses in their infant-directed than in their adult-directed speech (Fernald, 2001).

Infant-directed speech serves several purposes. The characteristic prosodic patterns of infant-directed speech appear to elicit infants' attention, modulate arousal, communicate affect, and facilitate language comprehension. First, with regard to eliciting attention, infants respond more to their own mother's voice when she is speaking in infant-directed tones than adult-directed tones. Infants also prefer to listen to infant-directed speech than to adult-directed speech even when spoken by strangers. Second, the sound and rhythm of infant-directed speech regulate infant state of arousal and communicate affect to the infant. Parents regularly coordinate their intonation with their communicative intent in specific contexts. American English, German, and Mandarin Chinese speaking mothers all use rising pitch contours to engage infant attention and elicit responses from an infant, falling contours to soothe a distressed infant, and up-and-down bell-shaped contours to maintain infant attention. Third, prosodic modifications of infant-directed speech facilitate infants' abilities to process speech and comprehend language. This exaggerated prosody helps infants meet the challenge of segmenting the speech stream and provides acoustic cues to the structure of linguistic messages. For example, infants discriminate speech sounds embedded in multisyllabic sequences better in streams of infant-directed speech than adult-directed speech.

No surprise, babies' brains are attuned to infant-directed speech. Within the first few months of life, infants neurologically process infant-directed speech differently from other auditory stimuli, and infant-directed speech of women (but not men) activates regions associated with reward in infants' frontal cortex (Naoi et al., 2012; Sulpizio et al., 2018).

Does infant-directed speech affect children's language development? One would think so, given all the foregoing evidence. But adults engage with infants in a number of verbal and nonverbal ways that help support language acquisition, and many of these activities occur together, so it is difficult to isolate the role of infant-directed speech *per se* from other behaviors, such as labeling (described next). Nevertheless, children whose onset of speech is delayed tend to have mothers who do not use exaggerated pitch in their speech.

LABELING

Parents often verbally refer to objects, activities, or events in the environment by labeling, describing, or asking about the unique qualities of the referent (*That's a spoon* and *What color is the dress?*). Using such referential language is reputedly associated with infants' acquiring vocabulary. Parents typically modify their speech to infants in different ways to enhance labeling. For example, labels have a high probability of being the loudest word in a sentence. The relative loudness of labels likely cues infants to map new words onto referent objects. Repetition is another common labeling strategy. For babies Dr. Seuss's *Mr. Brown can moo! Can you?* is a near perfect vehicle for repetition, for getting babies familiar with sounds, and for conveying that people and things have names. When parents use a name for a novel toy, they also exhibit a strong tendency to move the toy in synchrony with their verbal label, which may help infants make the association. The prosody of maternal speech is frequently linked to infants' object focus as well. But simple co-occurrence of a word and infants' attention to an object does not guarantee word learning. Social aspects of the situation facilitate linking word to object. For example, in one study infants who were exploring a novel toy heard an adult say, *A toma! It's a toma.* For some infants, the speaker was in view and was clearly talking to the infant. For other infants, the speaker was hidden behind a screen and had previously been seen talking on the telephone. Infants in the former condition learned that the object was a *toma.* By contrast, infants in the latter condition did not learn the word (Baldwin et al., 1996). This result is striking because, based on a simple association view of word learning, one would imagine that hearing a new word and simultaneously attending to a new toy would suffice for word learning, but this is not the case.

The amounts and types of speech parents use vary systematically with several sociodemographic characteristics of parents, such as their age, education, economic status, and ethnicity. Teen parents (and older siblings caring for younger siblings) talk less to infants than adult parents do, and across the early years the number of words children hear per hour differs dramatically by parent economic class: 616 words in families of the very poor, 1,251 in low-income families, and 2,153 in high-income families. These variations in input translate into variations in children's vocabulary, use of language, and language processing efficiency as early as children's second year. The amount of language input a child receives at 18 months also affects language processing speed and trajectories of vocabulary learning in English- and Spanish-learning children alike. Infants who received relatively more input at 18 months are faster in word recognition and know more words at 24 months (Hurtado et al., 2008).

Generally speaking, input matters. However, interpretation of the direction of influence is sometimes uncertain. It could be that parental speech influences infant speech *or* that infants who use nouns earlier promote the use of nouns by their parents. Still, infants with verbally responsive mothers enjoy larger vocabularies sooner and combine words into simple sentences earlier in their development than do infants with less verbally responsive mothers (see Box 4.4). Furthermore, experiments confirm the roles of experience. In one study, infants were taught invented verbs in transitive sentences, sentences with a direct object such as *The ball is dacking the car*, and in intransitive sentences, sentences with no direct object such as *The*

BOX 4.4   Set for Life? Language and Thought

How does language relate to thought? This question has also generated long-standing debate about the role that language may play in shaping cognition (Cook & Bassetti, 2011). Pruden and colleagues (2011) were interested in how parents' use of spatial language, as when they discuss object shapes and other properties, might impact their children's later spatial abilities. Fifty-two children and their caregivers were observed every 4 months from 19 months to 46 months of age while engaging in common daily activities. During these observations, the researchers noted the parents' and children's use of spatial language. At 54 months of age, children were assessed for their spatial understanding in three tasks. The researchers found wide variation in the extent to which parents use spatial language (range = 5 to 525 words) and similar variation in children's use of spatial language (range = 9 to 191 words). Moreover, parents who used a lot of spatial language had children who used a lot of spatial language. Parental spatial language use also predicted children's performance on tasks involving spatial transformation (e.g., select a shape that could be created from several pieces that are presented) and spatial analogies (e.g., select an abstract figure that preserves the spatial arrangement of a realistic picture). In short, what parents say may affect children's later cognition.

This discussion focuses on the values of parent speech to infants for infants. Language is fundamental to infant development, but also to the parent–infant relationship. Speech to babies is a major channel through which parents maintain contact ("I'll be right back."), interpret infants' cues ("Are you hungry again?") and respond to them ("Ok, let's try some peaches today."), introduce experiences ("Look at the pretty flower."), and express affection ("I love you so much!"). Parents who seldom speak to their babies forfeit a central means of connecting sensitively with their babies.

ball is dacking. Infants were then asked *What is the ball doing?* to see if they would use the verb transitively in new sentences (*Dacking the house*). Children who had been taught the verb in intransitive sentences almost never used it transitively (Brooks & Tomasello, 1998).

NONVERBAL SUPPORTS

In addition to using infant-directed speech and outright labeling, parents commonly (and unthinkingly) engage in many nonverbal strategies that support their infants' learning language. **Joint attention** occurs when two people attend to the same object. Bids for joint attention can be verbal, such as simply saying *Look!*; nonverbal, such as pointing; or verbal bids can be combined with nonverbal actions. Joint attention is not successful until the bid has been responded to. Responding to joint attention involves the partner acting on the verbal and/or nonverbal signal. Responses can be as simple as moving the eyes to where someone is pointing or looking. Given the limited action repertoire available to young infants, responding to joint attention appears earlier than initiating joint attention. Parents support joint attention in a number of ways. They introduce joint attention when they orient the focus of their infants' attention when infant are not already involved with an object; they maintain joint attention as when they follow and reinforce infants' focus of attention; and they redirect joint attention as when they change infants' ongoing focus of attention to a different object or topic. Engaging in joint attention allows infants to practice social attention management which is foundational to social interaction, and so joint attention also evidences the whole-child view of development.

Despite its value, not all children develop joint attention or are comfortable following others' eye gaze. Children diagnosed with autism spectrum disorder (ASD) appear to engage social and non social stimuli in relatively undifferentiated ways. Moreover, from observing home movies, researchers have noted that infants later diagnosed with ASD showed deficits in eye contact, pointing, and gaze monitoring. Luckily, training early in life can reduce some of the social deficits seen in infants diagnosed with ASD later in life.

Gaze following illustrates a successful response to a bid for joint attention. Remarkably, infants can follow a partner's gaze in the first few days after birth, but gaze following still develops across the first year. Initially, infants will follow head turns but only when an adults' eyes are open. Figure 4.3 shows an experimental set-up used to study gaze following. An adult and an infant are sitting across from each other, and on a table between them are two objects, one to their left and one to their right. The adult makes a head movement to look at one of the objects. On half of the trials the adult's eyes are

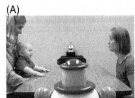 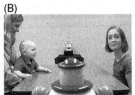 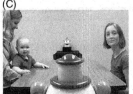

Figure 4.3 The sequence of events to assess gaze following. The experimenter (A) first makes eye contact with the infant then (B) looks at one of two objects. The infant shows successful gaze following by also looking at the object (C). (From Meltzoff & Brooks, 2009; reproduced with permission.)

open, and on the other half of the trials the adult's eyes are closed. Infants of 9 months follow the adult's head movement regardless of whether the adult's eyes are open or closed, and they overshoot the target, indicating that they may not be truly following the adult's gaze. Infants of 10 months demonstrate true gaze following by following the adult's head movements when the eyes are open but not when they are closed (Beier & Spelke, 2012). Gaze following is not unimportant in itself: Gaze following at 10½ months predicts vocabulary growth at 2½ years and understanding others' mental states at 4½ years.

Another type of non verbal communication between infant and caregiver that supports language learning is **gesture**. Gestures can be used to communicate information in the absence of language or enhance information in language. Pointing is a prominent gesture in communication. For example, a parent might point and at the same time ask the question *What is that?* or *Is that a ball?* or *Look! A ball*. For their part, infants are not only active in comprehending and speaking when they acquire language, they also use gestures. Long before the end of their first year, infants communicate about objects by reaching, giving, and showing. Everyone around infants will recognize that, even when they cannot say what they want, infants will find a way through their hands to "say" it anyway. In his diary, Darwin observed that his son Doddy regularly used gestures *to explain his wishes*. Perhaps the prototypical gesture for language-learning infants is pointing (Figure 4.4). Pointing by either the parent or the infant is an effective gesture for capturing a person's attention. Infants point a lot between 9 and 12 months of

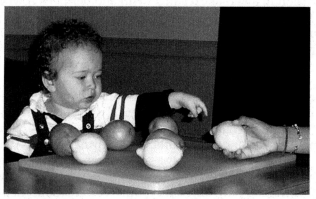

Figure 4.4 A child pointing during a categorization task. (Courtesy of M. Arterberry.)

age to indicate what they want. Over the course of the second year, infants use pointing in increasingly sophisticated ways, with older children pointing more when the other person does not appear to be looking at an interesting target. In addition, the appearance of pointing anticipates the emergence of language soon after.

Manual gestures are also common in the give and take of parent conversations with infants. Indeed, as formal language lags behind motor coordination in infant development, many infants resort to bodily movements of different kinds to convey their wants (everyone can envisage an infant seated with raised arms to indicate a desire to be picked up … no words necessary). Also' many parents successfully teach their infants hand "baby signs" for *milk, more, all done*, and the like.

TURN TAKING

Learning language is not a solitary endeavor but involves a social partner as well as pragmatic rules for engaging with that partner. Infants need to know sounds and words, certainly, but also how to interact with interlocutors, that is the people who take part in conversations. A number of rules govern social and verbal interactions. One important rule that is especially relevant to language is **turn taking**. Conversations proceed on the alternating give-and-take of one person holding the floor and then yielding to the other person. Adults conversing with one another regularly match timing factors in their speech. Turn taking is fundamental to the structure of adult dialogue. It is very difficult to both produce and process language at the same time. Almost everyone has been disconcerted on more than occasion in a verbal exchange with another person where you and they could not settle into an I-speak-and-you-listen-then-you-speak-and-I-listen format. It is also impolite to interrupt, so instead we wait our turn to speak.

Turn taking has deep roots in adult–infant exchanges. Long before infants produce formal speech, "proto-conversations" between parents and their infants involve a variety of alternating activities. For example, a nonverbal turn-taking "dialogue" quickly develops when mothers feed their newborns. When the infant pauses sucking, the mother moves the nipple. When the mother stops moving, the infant sucks again. From an extremely early age, infants produce different sounds, and their caregivers respond differently to different infant vocalizations depending on how caregivers interpret the sounds. When infants produce negative vocalizations, parents often respond by touching and talking to them. Moreover, infants produce more vocalizations when parents vocalize to them, rather than merely responding with a gesture. Reciprocal responding to vocalization is evident even in preterm infants.

Turn taking is equally a part of the basic games parents play with their infants. *Peek-a-boo* is an excellent example. In a typical scenario, the baby's face is covered with a blanket, a parent asks, *Where is [baby's name]?*, and then waits for the infant to remove the cloth. Once the cloth is removed, there is a period of shared joy (perhaps accompanied by the parent saying, *Oh … there you are!*). Older infants initiate the game by covering their own eyes and waiting for someone to ask "*Where is [baby's name]?*" Repetition of the game builds up an expectation of taking turns.

When infants start to vocalize, mothers and infants engage in alternating vocalizations, allowing both the chance to respond. One study recorded mothers interacting naturally at home and for 1 hour with their 5-month-olds in 11 different countries (Bornstein et al., 2015). Infants' non distress vocalizations and mothers' speech to infants were microcoded from the video/audio records, meaning that the onset and offset of each party's vocalization and speech bout were marked. Sequential analysis was then applied to the codings. In sequential analysis, the probability of a behavior is determined as a function of the occurrence of a previous behavior. The analytic rules asked for the probability of a mother beginning to speak to her infant within 2 seconds of her infant's stopping vocalizing, and reciprocally the probability of an infant beginning to vocalize within 2 seconds of the infant's mother stopping speech. In 9 of 11 countries, during an average hour together mothers were significantly likely to speak to their infant within 2 seconds of the infant stopping vocalizing, and in 5 of 11 counties infants were significantly likely to start vocalizing within 2 seconds of the end of their mothers speaking to them. From an early age, therefore, mothers and infants take turns in their verbal conversations.

Best practices for parents in conversation with their infants include vocalizing rapidly after an infant vocalization and using pauses after their own vocalizations to increase the likelihood that infant vocalizations will become part of a turn-taking conversational chain. For infants, this is an important first lesson in pragmatics (do not talk when someone else is talking). Infant vocalization is more likely to occur when a parent is present, and the amount of parent–preterm infant vocalization increases, suggesting that a conversational partner facilitates child language. This early and increasing propensity to engage in conversation in appropriate ways illustrates the extent to which infants are mainstreamed into a world of continual conversational turn taking.

Infants come to expect turn taking in many, if not all, of their interactions with others. This expectation is most notable in the **still-face paradigm**. This paradigm intentionally disrupts the normal course of interaction by asking an adult, typically the mother, to assume a "still face," that is not to respond to the normal vocal and social bids of her infant. This disruption fairly regularly leads to sadness and upset on the part of the infant. Infants expect call-and-response formats to verbal and social exchange. In fact, infants typically show more distress when the nonresponsive adult remains present in front of them than when the adult physically leaves the interaction altogether. As underscored in Chapter 3 in the discussion of infant memory, the salience of this disruption is evident in infants' negative reactions to the person involved in a still-face interaction over 1 year later (Bornstein et al., 2004).

MULTILINGUALISM

Infants growing up in the Global North are likely to live in societies dominated by a single language. Still, in many of those societies, a fifth to over a third of children do not solely hear a single language at home. By contrast, many societies in the Global South are multilingual which means that infants growing up there come into contact with more than one language as a normal part of everyday life. Although precise statistics are not available, it is likely that most infants today live in multilingual environments, and learning more than one language from birth (**multilingualism**) is increasingly the norm in much of the world (De Houwer, 2021).

Some multilingual environments provide balanced input of two or more languages. In these cases, often one parent speaks one language and the other parent speaks a second language, or there is a public national language and one or more personal (family or tribal) languages. Infants exposed from birth to two languages may eventually speak one or the other or both languages. In other cases, infants' parents may speak a language in the home that is different from the dominant language or parents may not even be fluent in the dominant language of the society. This latter example characterizes the context for infants in many immigrant families, and in this context it is often hard to maintain the minority language once children go to school and interact with peers. Social interaction is important for learning language, and children quickly learn which language is dominant in their wider community.

In contexts where infants hear equal amounts of input from two languages, there is only a small amount of confusion between the two languages, and infants tend to achieve language development milestones around the same ages as infants learning only one language. In comparison to monolinguals, bilingual infants may have smaller vocabularies in each language; however, their vocabulary in the two languages (when counting unique words) is equal in size to that of monolinguals. As is true of monolinguals, how many words in a given language a bilingual infant knows or says likely reflects that infant's exposure to the two languages. Infants exposed to more than one language acquire vocabulary in each language at levels that generally match the ratio of exposure to one language versus another. In other words, an infant whose linguistic environment is predominantly Spanish with some English will speak more Spanish words than English words (Figure 4.5).

These accomplishments are impressive when we stop to consider all that infants need to do when they hear two languages. The 4 (domains of language) × 2 (comprehension and production) achievements described earlier in this chapter and shown in

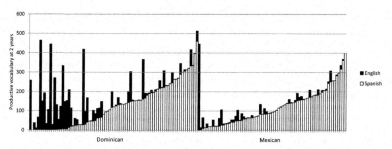

Figure 4.5 Productive vocabulary in English and Spanish of 2-year-olds of Mexican and Dominican heritage. Each bar shows an individual child. There is variability in the proportion of English versus Spanish words each child produces, an effect attributed to the frequency of each language the child hears in the home. (From Song et al., 2012; Copyright © 2012 by the American Psychological Association. Reproduced with permission. The use of APA information does not imply endorsement by APA.)

	Phonology	Semantics	Syntax	Pragmatics
Comprehension				
Production				

Figure 4.6 The language domain matrix for acquiring more than one language. (Created by M. H. Bornstein.)

Figure 4.1 is multiplied by 2 (or more languages) since learning two languages is at least as (or more) challenging than 1 + 1 (Figure 4.6). Infants are hearing two different sound systems and extracting regularities of each. They also need to preserve their abilities to perceive important sound contrasts across the two languages. They are determining the statistical regularities of each language, such that they can find boundaries for syllables, words, and phrases. Furthermore, they are learning that the same object can have two names (like *dog* in English and *chien* in French). Finally, they need to learn different grammatical rules for parts of speech and word order (for example, subject-verb-object in English, but subject-object-verb in Korean). Although some pragmatics likely spill over from one language to another (e.g., turn taking), other pragmatic rules may differ (as making eye contact with an interlocutor which is expected in some cultures but discouraged in others). The overall result is complex mental and vocal representations of two (or more) languages.

An important consequence of this diversity is the large variability in multilingualism. One example study assessed language in infants from two Latin American immigrant groups in the United States. The two differed significantly in their productive and receptive vocabularies and language dominance, and they displayed strengths in different areas of communication. For example, Mexican American infants had larger receptive vocabularies at 14 months of age, and Dominican American infants had larger productive vocabularies at 24 months of age (Song et al., 2012).

It is widely believed today that bilingual children enjoy certain cognitive advantages even outside of communication. Some developmental psycholinguists posit that the flexibility required for using two languages spills over into positive effects in speed of processing information and imitation. Whether or not there are such spill-over effects from learning more than one language from birth, there is tremendous value in being able to speak and understand more than one language. Language is for communicating with others, and bilingual children are doubly prepared for this task. Indeed, as their dual mental representations develop, children may engage in **code-switching**, inserting words from one language while speaking another language. Code-switching is a natural process of development, and something that multilingual adults readily and often do. Code-switching does not mean confusing two languages; code-switching is the result of knowing the word in one language but not the other, or knowing a better fitting phrase in one language than the other. Code-switching is an example of how multilingualism illustrates cognitive flexibility.

A final word about infant multilingualism. Most of what is known about language development – the information that has filled this chapter – was gleaned from infants growing up monolingually. It is likely that the course of bilingual child language development is similar to monolingual child language development in broad strokes. But as multilingualism outpaces monolingualism in the world, we should be prepared to revise our understanding of how infants become effective communicators.

SUMMARY

From its Latin roots, infancy literally means incapable of speech, yet this period of life contains the foundations for and the first steps toward language acquisition and proficiency. Infants learn only the particular language (and even the idiosyncratic dialect) to which they are exposed, and individual differences and individual experiences are associated with remarkable variation in infants' eventual language competencies. Comprehension generally precedes production, and communication begins well before infants' first words emerge – via babbling, gestures, and the like. The appearance of first words constitutes a significant milestone, likely representing a cognitive revolution in infants' understanding of what language is and what it is used for. How infants learn words is still debated, but both nature and nurture doubtlessly have their say. On the one hand, infants must rely on natural constraints to help with this process. On the other hand, and happily, parents readily adjust the language they direct to their infants in multiple ways that appear to support their infants' task, and numerous supports in the infant's linguistic environment facilitate language learning. In the end, infant language acquisition must be both rigid and flexible. Rigid in the sense that infant language acquisition must assure desired outcomes even in the face of experiential diversity and instability. Flexible in the sense that infant language acquisition needs to be responsive to specific experiences with the specific language they will acquire. The marvel is that, however complex and challenging language is, infants make great progress in understanding language and communicating with language even before they can tie their shoes and without much, if any, formal instruction.

5

FEELING

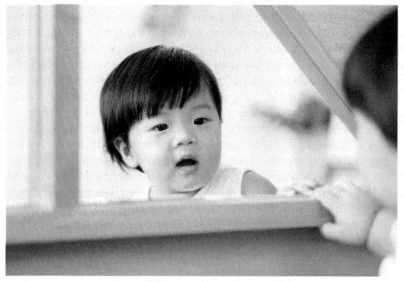

(Image courtesy of Shutterstock, copyright: Hua_khai/Shutterstock.com.)

INTRODUCTION

Just as infants are growing, thinking, and communicating beings, they are feeling beings as well. By "feeling" we mean that infants express their own emotions and respond to emotions in others, that

DOI: 10.4324/9781003172802-5

infants have temperaments which are presumptive of a future personality, and that infants are rapidly developing a sense of themselves. Feelings involve emotions, temperament, and self, the three subjects of this *Basics* chapter.

Everyone around infants notices their emotions, both positive and negative. Indeed, most everyone who interacts with infants works hard to elicit and track infants' expressions of emotions and their emotional development. Consider just three expressions that mark emotional milestones of infant development: their first smiles, the earliest indications of stranger wariness, and initial signs of embarrassment. These emotional reactions are also significant because parents view them as indicators of children's state and what parents must respond to. Infants' temperament in believed to reveal cues to the children's emerging personality – what their children's behavioral style is like now and what they might be like in future years.

Emotions and temperament have several features in common. Each has a long and contentious history of theory and study, each is notoriously difficult to pin down in definition, each significantly influences infants' immediate as well as lasting relationships with other people, each filters and colors infants' experiences, and each is a fundamental constituent of the self, or who we are. For these reasons, these two realms of "feeling" are notoriously slippery and difficult to disentangle. Very roughly speaking, emotions are fleeting feelings whether they are generated internally (as by thoughts) or externally (as by experiences); a baby's sudden and unexpected cower at the sight of a strange mechanical toy may illustrate a passing emotional response of fear. By contrast, temperament is thought of as a more consistent core of acting and reacting to experiences and the environment; a baby who has an easy temperament may find the same strange mechanical toy interesting and seek to explore it. By temperament, this child also is likely to be regular in feeding, hardly frets when being put to sleep, accommodates to new experiences, and responds warmly to strangers.

This chapter treats infants' emotions, temperament, and self separately, but the whole child is a bundle of interrelated emotions embedded in a burgeoning style of temperament that together construct a self. The self is an even more challenging construct that we address in the third part of the chapter. Newborns do not give any evidence that they know who they are or even that they exist. It turns out that children recognizing that they exist as separate entities is fairly difficult to prove in any definitive way. Yet, developmental scientists have found means to tap into infants' psyches to converge on a recognizable developmental timetable. Knowing that we are and who we are, different facets of a self, is key in many ways to who we become.

EMOTIONS

To get our arms around what emotions are in infancy and what meaning they have to infants and to those around them, we have to consider separate constituents of emotions from listing emotions, defining emotions, and measuring emotions finally to understanding the development of emotional expressions in infants and infants' responses to emotional expressions in others. Developmental scientists are interested in explaining how changes in emotional expression and emotional sensitivity emerge and develop.

Emotions help to organize infants' responses. Individual differences in predominant mood, soothability, and intensity characterize infants' emotions. Parents (and developmental scientists) pay especially close attention to infants' emotions because emotions color infants' encounters with the social and inanimate world. Asked to describe the range of emotions they naturally perceive in their babies, 99% of mothers of 1-month-olds profess that their babies express interest, 95% joy, 84% anger, 75% surprise, 58% fear, and 34% sadness. Parents increasingly characterize their infants by their emotional expressions, and paying attention to infants' emotional reactions helps parents to manage, pacify, accentuate, or direct infant development effectively.

The study of emotions and emotional development poses fundamental questions for the measurement and interpretation of infant behavior. In this section, we consider these questions, starting with the definition of emotion.

PRIMARY AND SECONDARY EMOTIONS

What developmental scientists today consider an emotion depends heavily on how they define emotions, and it is hardly surprising that different developmental scientists, just as their philosopher forebears, have defined emotions in radically different ways. That is, different scholars of emotions have produced distinctive lists. One way in which emotions have been distinguished is by contrasting primary with secondary emotions. Primary emotions are asserted to be deeply rooted in human biology, and thus are either innate or very quickly developing. Although there is disagreement about just what all the primary emotions are, most authorities would include: interest, joy, surprise, sadness, anger, disgust, fear, and shyness. In contrast, secondary emotions are less biological in origin and tend to reflect later developmental achievements. Secondary emotions emerge during the second and third years of life as the capacities for self-referential thought and appraisal develop. Secondary emotions include embarrassment, pride, guilt, shame, and envy.

DEFINING INFANT EMOTIONS

Like most other BIG concepts in psychology – intelligence, personality – definitions of emotion have defied easy consensus. Take the seemingly simple case of a baby smile. We see the smile and (of course!) want to believe that it signals a state of internal happiness in that LO, and (of course!) the thing we did or even our mere presence elicited the smile and that state of internal happiness. But who is to say that a facial expression reliably reflects an underlying emotion? (And who has not been corrected that a baby's smile is just gas?) Similarly, does the baby's capacity to see my facial expression in any way reflect the baby's understanding of emotions?

One popular approach to defining emotions analyses them in terms of their component processes, their *structure* so to speak. For example, developmental scientists in the emotions business propose that emotions have (at least) five essential structural components:

1. Emotions have a biological basis, and so-called emotion elicitors are external or internal events that trigger emotional reactions.
2. There are corresponding emotion receptors in the brain that register and encode emotion-relevant events.
3. Emotion states involve biological activity activated by emotion receptors.
4. Facial, gestural, and other behaviors express emotions.
5. The interpretation and evaluation of perceived emotional states and expressions constitute emotional experience.

From this definition of emotions, emotional life incorporates biology, cognition, and sociality (growing, thinking, and relating in the whole-child perspective). On the one hand, this approach to emotions has value because it throws light on biological and cognitive influences underlying emotional reactions. Insofar as developing mental processes are involved, for example, it must be that infants of various ages evaluate and interpret emotional cues in different ways and so appraise emotions differently. On the other hand, focusing on components and underlying processes underestimates or neglects reciprocal influences emotions exert on other aspects of development. Emotions are richer than just being the by-product of biological or cognitive processes; they also influence perception, cognition, and sociability.

An alternative approach to understanding emotions emphasizes their *functions* in everyday life as opposed to focusing on components of their structure. Emotions are adaptive and have uses in ongoing interactions between people and their environments. In this sense, people apply emotions intentionally to communicate states or facts with others and to achieve certain goals. Emotions constitute cues that can cause an individual to evaluate their current circumstances in one or another way (as when fear prompts flight), just as emotions provide cues to others about an individual's current state or how others are to respond to the individual (to comfort a sad face). From this functionalist view, emotions shape relations between the individual and a context. Consider the several ways in which emotions do what they do. Emotions influence perception, cognition, and motivation and in doing so cause people to re-evaluate their current condition and adjust their actions accordingly. Emotions influence how people appraise and interpret events and how they organize their experiences conceptually. Emotions can also regulate interpersonal behavior because individuals respond socially to the emotions they read in others and adjust their emotional expressions to achieve their social goals. The approach of someone who is visibly angry (with clenched fists, a flushed face, and an irate facial expression) arouses different emotions and reactions than the approach of someone who looks joyful or fearful.

Finally, emotions organize and motivate reactions to environmental events that may be biologically and/or psychologically adaptive. Compare, for example, the goals, action tendencies, and adaptive functions of joy versus anger. People express joy when they conclude that significant objectives or goals have been attained, and these emotional experiences energize them, reinforcing activity, encouraging others to maintain the pleasurable interaction, and stimulating them to attempt new challenges. By contrast, people express anger when they perceive obstacles that prevent them from attaining their goals. Anger motivates efforts to restore progress toward achieving the goal, changing the behavior of others, and/or striving for revenge or retaliation. The functionalist orientation regards emotions as central organizing features of human experience. It recognizes that emotions are influenced by biology and cognition but also emphasizes the purposes of emotions. In some respects, these two views of emotion – the structuralist view and the functionalist view – differ in emphases rather than substance. The two explain identical emotional processes in complementary ways.

ORIGINS AND DEVELOPMENT OF INFANT EMOTIONS

Where do emotions come from, why are some emotions positive and others negative, and do emotions change with age? The developmental scientist Watson theorized that infants learn three basic emotions – love, fear, rage – through classical conditioning (Chapter 3). In this view, neutral stimuli (the CS of a mother's voice or face) that are paired with unconditioned stimuli (the UCS of warmth or food) that elicit an unconditioned emotional response (a UCR of happiness) become conditioned stimuli that elicit the same positive emotions (the CR). Similarly, operant conditioning and observational learning have been invoked to account for the origins of infant emotions. Infants' smiles are likely rewarded by adult caregivers who smile back and also provide opportunities for infants to observe and imitate smiling and other emotional expressions (like surprise). These modes of learning seem intuitive and powerful explanations for how and why infants acquire emotional associations and increase or decrease their expressions of emotion. Curiously, however, learning theories do not explain why emotional reactions first occur. Babies start to smile at about 6 weeks of age, but they have been fed, held, caressed, and smiled at before then. Also, babies who are blind from birth begin to smile at the same age as sighted infants, so imitation might be an unlikely source of emotional learning.

Psychodynamic theorists proposed similar experiential origins of emotions. Rene Spitz (1887–1974), an Austrian-American psychoanalyst, believe that emotions partly grew out of parent–infant interaction. Similar to learning theory, parents' actions shape infants' emotions as parents positively gratify infants' physical needs (hunger). These positive emotions simultaneously lend parents a special positive significance. To instill self-control (say, to restrict children from crawling/falling down stairs), parents must also frustrate children, and in doing so they elicit negative emotions. So, the particular configuration of parental facial features, involving the forehead, eyes, and nose, comes to elicit a corresponding facial expression in babies. However, psychoanalytic theories have difficulties in explaining some aspects of infant emotional development. For example, psychoanalytic theories are constructed around parent–infant relationships, but infants respond emotionally not just to parents. Young infants also respond emotionally to a variety of other stimuli. Infants smile at bull's-eye patterns and pets; older infants show fear to heights, masks, and jack-in-the-box toys.

Contrasting learning and psychodynamic theories of emotion are ethological and evolutionary ones that emphasize biological or maturational determinants of infant emotional life. As noted above, smiling emerges in infants (even infants blind from birth) at approximately 6 weeks of age as if following a maturational time-table, independent of any social experiences. Moreover, some emo-tional expressions are culturally universal. This universality across infant ability and cultural context leads ethologists to conclude that emotions play a role in ensuring survival. **Ethology** is the scientific study of animal behavior. Rhesus monkeys (a close evolutionary cousin to humans) raised in isolation nevertheless respond with fear to pictures of other monkeys in threatening postures. Because these monkeys have never had an opportunity to learn the emotion, the conclusion is that certain emotions may have innate, biologi-cal bases. Evolutionary psychology interprets maturational, species similar, and culturally universal adaptive findings as indicators of species survival and useful toward reproductive success (ensuring continuation of the genes). For example, happy and sad expressions both bring caring adults closer, which contribute to the well-being of the baby. Yet, it is not always the case that infant emotions serve an adaptive purpose. Infants do not innately fear snakes or spiders, even though it is adaptive to do so.

Infant expressions of emotion and underlying emotional experi-ences also develop over time through nervous system maturation and social experience into a differentiated emotional repertoire. Rounding out a whole-child view of infant emotional life, per-ception and cognition appear to be essential to infant emotions. Whether infants display a positive or negative emotional reaction to a stimulus, say a stranger, might depend, among other things, on the context in which the stimulus is encountered. Infants respond more positively to strangers in familiar circumstances (such as at home) than in unfamiliar ones (such as a pediatrician's office). Friendliness toward strangers is also more apparent when strangers approach slowly and gradually rather than suddenly and abruptly, and when the mother or another trusted adult reacts positively to the stranger in front of the child. Thus, the strangeness of the unfamiliar adult does not by itself determine the emotional reaction. Rather, the con-text and manner in which the stranger is encountered (hence the infants' cognitive interpretation) influence whether infants emote a positive (sociable) or negative (frightened) reaction.

STUDYING INFANT'S EMOTIONS SCIENTIFICALLY

How can we ever know what someone else is really feeling ... especially if that someone else is an infant? One thing going for us is that, unlike adults, infants do not hide their feelings. It could be, then, that infants' feelings are an open book. A smile is a smile, and a cry is a cry ... period. Still, the fact that infants cannot describe their subjective experiences of emotions to us presents an obstacle to genuinely understanding emotions and emotional development in infancy. The best that developmental scientists have done is to study emotional sensitivity and emotional expression (even though expressions might not always reflect sensitivity very well) and knit the two together to tell a story.

In his 1872 book on *The Expression of the Emotions in Man and Animals*, Darwin focused on facial expressions of emotion, noting that certain expressions are remarkably consistent across age and culture. The face has 42 muscles that can be used to express emotions; adults commonly use all of them to express emotions, and adults primarily evaluate someone else's emotions by relying on their face. On the twin principles of cephalocaudal and proximodistal development, from an early age infants also command muscles in their face to express their emotions. Little wonder that developmental scientists have also looked to the face to assess emotions in infants.

Two developmental science approaches have prevailed to study emotions formally. One is to code facial muscles and their movements based on detailed anatomical measurement systems. These systems have been used to speculate when specific emotions are being experienced and to track developmental change in emotion expression. For example, advances in videorecording technology slow down otherwise fleeting real-life experiences to reveal levels of detail in emotional expression otherwise easily missed. Not to put too fine a point on it (and scientists cannot help themselves in doing so), this kind of approach has parsed infant smiles into four distinct types (Figure 5.1): (1) simple smiling: smiling involving neither cheek raising nor mouth opening, (2) Duchenne smiling: cheek-raised smiling without mouth opening, (3) play smiling: open-mouth smiling without cheek raising, and (4) duplay smiling: open-mouth cheek-raised smiling.

Emotion has physiological components as well, and developmental scientists have tapped into infant physiological states to index emotion. Changes in skin temperature (as when infants begin to laugh) provide unique information regarding emotional experience.

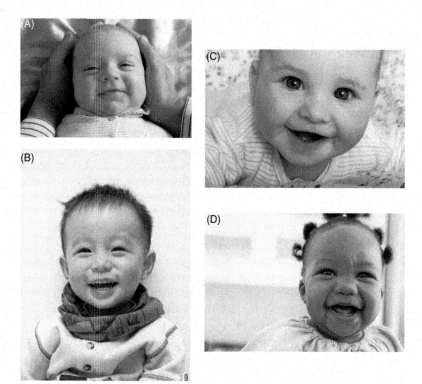

Figure 5.1 Examples of four different types of smiles: (A) simple smile; (B) Duchenne smile; (C) play smile; and (D) duplay smile. (Images courtesy of Shutterstock.com, copyright: Vira Mylyan-Monastyrska/Shutterstock.com, qingqing/Shutterstock.com, Jirik V/Shutterstock.com, Monkey Business Images/Shutterstock.com.)

After 4 months of age, laughing is accompanied by a decrease in skin temperature, particularly around the nose (Nakanishi & Imai-Matsumura, 2008).

To adult observers, infants' facial expressions seem to clearly signal joy, anger, fear, and other discrete primary emotions. But still, interpretation calls for a leap of faith. As hinted earlier, facial expression may not accurately indicate infants' underlying emotional experience, and infants do not always show the same facial expression in the same situation.

The face is a natural place to start, but other bodily systems signal emotions as well. Voice as well as posture, gesture, and movement can all express emotion. Adult speech that has high pitch, pitch variability, fast tempo, and high intensity is associated with happiness, whereas low pitch, low intensity, slow tempo, and diminished pitch variability in adult speech are associated with sadness. Infants cry for different reasons – hunger, pain, sleepiness, and frustration, for example – and infants cry in distinct ways indicating hunger versus pain, a sound difference evident to most caregivers. Certain cries impress adults as more distressed and aversive than others. For example, high-pitched, intense, long-lasting cries are heard to indicate greater distress and consequently elicit quicker responses from adults. Age is also a factor in cry. Younger infants cry more (on average about 3 hours per day); older infants cry less. Also, the acoustic features of infant cries change as infants mature, in part due to anatomical changes in the growing vocal tract.

With respect to posture, gesture, and movement, infants become very still when they appear to be especially interested in something, they turn away from stimuli that appear to evoke fear, slump in posture when they appear to be sad, and exhibit excitement as if trying to repeat or duplicate experiences that appear to elicit joy (Figure 5.2). Posture, gesture, and movement may not be associated with different emotions in a one-to-one fashion, but they offer useful information when connected to facial and/or vocal indicators of infant emotions.

In addition to direct observations of infant emotions as just described, mothers and others (nurses, students) have been enlisted to identify infants' emotions. Identification of emotions by such untrained observers is still fairly accurate for some emotional expressions (interest, joy, surprise) but less so for others (anger, fear, shyness). Mothers report that they typically base their judgments of their infants' emotions on facial and vocal cues, along with gestures and arm movements. Whether these judgments accurately reflect infants' expressive capacities or mothers' subjective inferences based on contextual cues or both is not known. Certainly, mothers respond differently to different perceived emotions, an ability that likely arises from their accruing experiences and feedback from their babies.

Despite these advances, the study of infant emotions is clearly challenging. Developmental scientists have devised several ways to measure infants' emotional expressions. However, distinguishing among some infant emotional expressions (as telling anger and fear apart) is no easy matter, and physiological indicators do not always match infants' measured emotional expressions. As with evaluations of other structures and functions in infancy, reliance on any single index of emotional arousal in infants – whether facial,

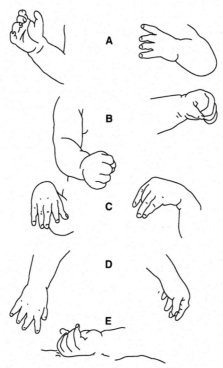

Figure 5.2 Observable cues indicating behavioral and emotional states of infants as seen in the position of hands: (A) alert waking state, (B) closed fists in a distressed state, (C) passive waking, (D) transition to sleep, and (E) sleep. (Courtesy of H. Papoušek.)

vocal, or postural – is dicey and risks arriving at erroneous or biased conclusions. As with other areas of infancy, developmental science has learned the value of using multiple convergent measures when studying infants' emotions.

DEVELOPMENT OF INFANTS' EMOTIONAL EXPRESSIONS

Just as there are two sides to communicating (comprehending and producing language), emotional competence has two sides, one that involves expressing emotions and one that involves reading others' emotions. Infant development involves both. Here we look at infants' production and comprehension of emotions in broad strokes.

Emotional expressions spring in part from biologically adaptive actions, so it is not surprising that even newborns might be capable of expressing some primary emotions. Developmental scientists who study emotional development have documented some neonatal expressions of emotions, which seem to relate to deeply seated survival-related experiences. For example, nutritious foods are to be ingested, and noxious ones avoided. So, it is telling that newborns respond to sweet tastes (banana) and odors (vanilla) with positive facial expressions and to bitter tastes (vinegar) and foul odors (rotten eggs) with negative expressions (Figure 1.7). However, newborns seem capable of only a limited range of primary emotional expressions, and emotional expressiveness certainly becomes more differentiated with age.

Infants express both positive and negative emotions. The earliest elicited smiles to another person's voice or face appear around 6 weeks of age. Clear expressions of joy have been observed by 2½ months when infants are playing with their mothers, and by 3 to 4 months of age infants will laugh in response to social stimulation that is more arousing and intense. Joy also occurs in non social situations. Infants show more joy and interest in contingent games (peek-a-boo) than noncontingent games.

Among primary negative emotions, infants also express unhappiness facially and vocally from birth. An observational study of infants in each of two cultural groups in each of five countries (Argentina, Belgium, Israel, Italy, and the United States) revealed that 5-month-olds in all groups all displayed unhappiness via facial and vocal cues in approximately equal amounts during an average hour in the day (Bornstein, 2022). With maturation and experience, generalized unhappiness later differentiates into sadness, disgust, fear, and anger. By itself, anger becomes increasingly typical in response to events that are unpleasant or physically restricting. For example, distress predominates as the emotional response of 2-month-olds to painful inoculations, but it is replaced by anger at 19 months. Likewise, when mothers play with their 2- or 3-month-old infants and then suddenly become unresponsive (the still-face procedure), their babies show signs of withdrawal, wariness, and sadness in their faces and postures. It is noteworthy that infants react in much the same way when their social partner looks at a mobile phone, rather than being responsive to them. The status of certain emotions (e.g., fear) is less certain. On the one hand, 6- to 9-month-old infants show no fear of snakes, one of the most feared stimuli across all humanity. On the other hand, infants as young as 6 weeks of age respond defensively to a fast-approaching or looming object (as described in in Chapter 3). An infant's reflexive eye blink might not be a full-blown emotional expression of fear, but it likely anticipates that very same reaction to threat in adults.

Infants' social experiences help to shape their emotional expressiveness. Mothers' facial expressions change an average of seven to nine times per minute during face-to-face play with their infants. Roughly one-quarter of the time, mothers respond promptly to their infants' expressions, typically by imitating or responding positively to positive expressions, especially those of younger infants, and just as often ignoring negative expressions. As their infants grow into the second half of their first year, mothers are increasingly responsive to their infants' positive expressions (interest, joy). Not surprisingly, infants also increase their expressiveness over this period, displaying more positive emotions.

Emotional expressiveness in mothers and infants tends to resemble one another. It is possible that familial similarities in emotional expressiveness reflect the genetics that parents and their infants share (nature). However, parents also socialize their infants' emotions by expressing certain emotions themselves which infants can see and imitate and by responding to infants in ways that accord with individual proclivities and cultural norms and expectations of emotional expressiveness (nurture). In this perspective, infants' emotional displays are socialized through infants' emotionally resonant or empathic responses to parents' emotional states. Darwin wrote that, when only 6 months old, his son Doddy seemed to express sympathy when the boy's nurse pretended to cry. Pre-empathic capacities appear very early in life in a form of **emotional contagion** whereby a baby spontaneously resonates with another baby's emotional expression, most often observed in response to distress. In a circumstance well known to nurses in newborn nurseries, one infant's cry can set off other infants to cry (Sagi & Hoffman, 1976). It is easy to see how such responses might anticipate or even transmute into genuine empathy.

Atypical circumstances of development also reveal a lot about infants' emotional lives. Parents can foster affective disturbance in infants through socialization. Pregnancy and childbirth are well-known risk factors for maternal depression. In the United States, perhaps 13% of women experience symptoms of depression, and globally many new mothers reportedly experience depression symptoms and disorders. Importantly, maternal depression is associated with negative parenting cognitions and harsh and withdrawn parenting practices which can disrupt mother–infant interactions. Infants of depressed mothers show depressed social behaviors (withdrawn, immobile, and non responsive) when interacting with their mothers that spills over to interactions with strangers. Infants may acquire such socioemotional styles through genetic transmission, by imitating their mothers' behavior, as psychological effects of maternal depression, or all of the above. It is well established that infants of depressed mothers display more negative affect, but other experiences can also shape one's emotional life, as the sobering example in Box 5.1 illustrates.

BOX 5.1   Set for Life? The Effects of Experience on Perception of Emotions

Do early experiences affect how infants perceive and respond to emotional expressions? Infants recognize different facial expressions that characterize a range of emotions. Pollak and colleagues (2009) discovered that overexposure to certain emotions affects how children perceive certain emotions but not others. Nine-year-olds viewed five emotional expressions posed by different models that ranged in intensity and were asked to say if the model looked happy, afraid, angry, surprised, or showed no emotion. Children who had been physically abused by their parents identified less intense angry expressions as angry compared to well-treated children. When identifying happiness, surprise, and fear, the abused and well-treated children performed similarly. Likely children who are abused experience expressions of anger more often than well-treated children and so may be more sensitive to earlier displays of anger.

The first year of life may be a sensitive period for perceiving different emotional displays. Camras and colleagues (2006) explored this possibility by taking advantage of a natural experiment: In many Chinese and Eastern European orphanages, children experience emotional and social deprivation. Their study compared perceptions of emotions among Chinese and Eastern European 4- to 5-year-old children who had been adopted. The Eastern European children experienced 16½ months of institutionalized care on average, whereas the Chinese children experienced only 8 months of institutionalized care. Children were tested in two tasks. One task involved hearing stories about an emotional situation, after which children were asked to identify the appropriate emotion. The second task involved emotion-labeling, and children were asked to select from four facial expressions the one that matched an emotional label, such as "happy." Eastern European children performed worse on both tasks compared to the Chinese children, a difference possibly attributable to the different lengths of time children spent in institutionalized care in the first years of life.

Support for this interpretation comes from a study with infants. Infants of depressed mothers process facial expressions differently from those of well mothers. Bornstein and colleagues (2011) used the habituation-test paradigm to compare infants' discrimination of a smiling and a neutral expression.

Infants of depressed and well mothers habituated to the repeated presentation of a facial stimulus with a given expression in the same way, suggesting that infants in both groups process information similarly. However, infants of depressed mothers showed no evidence that they could distinguish a smiling from a neutral face, whereas infants of well mothers made the distinction. Thus, the experience of having a depressed mother who smiles infrequently, if at all, seems to have affected infants' perceptions and responsiveness to facial expressions.

As infancy proceeds and infants achieve self-awareness, self-conscious secondary emotions, such as embarrassment, pride, guilt, and shame emerge. As described later in this chapter, an index of infants' self-awareness is their recognizing themselves in a mirror. Infants 15 to 24 months of age who recognize themselves in a mirror also look embarrassed when they are effusively praised by an adult: They smile and look away, cover their faces with their hands, and the like. Infants who do not recognize themselves do not respond in this way to adult praise. The emergence of self-awareness also fosters a better understanding of emotions.

Thus, infants can express a range of primary positive and negative emotions across a range of situations from the first months of life. As infants grow older, they express an increasingly widening range of emotions and are emotionally responsive to a growing variety of situations. Developmental scientists today believe that neural maturation facilitates the expression of more complex secondary emotions and renders possible the inhibition of negative emotions. Infants' cognitive development also contributes to emotional growth by enabling infants to evaluate the meaning of different situations. For example, infants' reactions to strangers at the end of the first year call on their evaluation of an approaching adult (as familiar or unfamiliar) as well as the context (whether mother is present or not), the setting (a comfortable and familiar or unfamiliar environment), the stranger's appearance (whether male or female, child or adult), and behavior (approaching fast or slow, looming overhead or looking at eye level). The fact that infants' emotional expressiveness is bound up with their physiology, perception, and cognition amply confirms the whole-child view of infancy. Their maturing physiology along with their growing mental skills underlie infants' increasingly sophisticated appraisals of themselves, their situations, and their experiences that in turn underlie their emotional reactions. In other words, greater sophistication in thoughts and emotions go hand in hand. Additionally, infants' accruing language skills make possible alternative forms of emotional expression so infants can "use their words" – rather than cries or clenched fists – to express their emotions.

DEVELOPMENT OF INFANTS' SENSITIVITY TO OTHERS' EMOTIONAL EXPRESSIONS

Being sensitive to emotional expressions involves reading and adjusting to them as well as sending appropriate emotional signals in return. Many developmental scientists have studied infants' growing capacities to read facial expressions as cues to emotions in others. However, discriminating different facial expressions is not the same as understanding their meaning, and thus "reading" emotions requires sophisticated interpretive as well as basic perceptual capacities. Because visual acuity in early infancy is limited, newborns are likely limited in distinguishing among different facial features and expressive patterns. Starting by around 1½ to 2 months of age, infants can discriminate among different facial expressions, and by 5 months they even distinguish among and categorize variations in the intensity of some emotional expressions (Figure 3.7). Again, these achievements do not mean that these infants *understand* emotional meaning in facial expressions. Infants may just be responding differently to different facial configurations (e.g., eyebrow position or mouth open or closed) without ascribing any specific emotional values to them.

Healthy infants appear to become more genuinely emotionally responsive to facial expressions between 4 and 9 months of age. Infants in this age range can match their own expressions to the emotional expressions of adults, and they may even be learning more enduring socioemotional styles from their caregivers. Other related developments in this period support this conclusion. For example, at this time infants begin to respond differently to different vocal correlates of emotional expressions and begin to coordinate vocal and facial features of emotional expressions. Infants also show differential neural processing to positive and negative emotional expressions. Moreover, infants' scanning of threat-related facial expressions, such as fear and anger, develops across the middle of the first year, as they increasingly avoid looking at eyes. In short, as infants grow older and achieve perceptual sophistication in discriminating faces and cognitive sophistication in categorization, they begin to take others' emotional expressions into account more comprehensively.

Around 8 to 9 months of age, infants appear to appreciate that others' emotional expressions pertain to specific objects or events. Indeed, around this age infants use others' emotional expressions to help them understand (particularly ambiguous) situations. **Social referencing** is a term used to refer to infants' deliberate search for information to help clarify uncertain or novel events. For example, infants may not approach a novel and ambiguous object unless a trusted adult indicates that it is ok to do so by smiling or otherwise providing positive signals (Schmitow & Stenberg, 2013; Stenberg, 2017). Similarly, infants stop playing with unusual toys when their mothers show disgust as opposed to pleasure, and they continue to avoid such toys even after their mothers stop posing distinct emotional expressions and are instead silent and neutral. Infants also reference emotional information presented by televised models. As well, children's peers are recognized as sources of emotional information, but not until around 24 months, and infants retain information gained in social referencing for surprisingly long times. In short, facial and vocal expressions of emotion assume intensifying significance for infants. This development is hardly surprising. Emotional expressions are among humanity's most important social signals, and thus we should expect that babies are attuned to them early in life. As infants proceed through their second year, their social competence and sensitivity are fostered, in part, by their enhanced sophistication at reading the emotions of others.

Emotions are fleeting transitory feelings, usually reactions to people, objects, or events. Temperaments are considered more permanent or generalized styles of reactivity. Of course, a sudden loud sound or the precipitous invasion of a stranger into an infant's personal space may set the most temperamentally easy-going baby to react negatively. However, some babies are prone to react positively or negatively almost always and across many different situations on accounts of their differing temperaments.

TEMPERAMENT

Infants, like adults, have identifiable individual behavioral styles of responding to experiences and the environment. We describe some specific styles in a moment, but need to set the stage and discuss these styles more generally first. Developmental scientists refer to such individual styles as **temperament**. Because individual temperamental styles appear so early in life, they are thought to originate in genetics and the biology of the infant. However, the fact that temperament is rooted in genetics and biology does not necessarily mean that temperament is fixed and immutable; influences of genetics change over time, and experiences shape genetics and the expression of temperament.

Reinforcing these notions, temperaments tend to be stable over person, situation, and time. A temperamentally "sociable" infant is likely to manifest sociability consistently even with different people, in different situations, and at different times and ages. Sociable infants smile and reach out and later as sociable children approach and easily engage with other people.

Infants express their temperaments by their behaviors. When thinking about temperamental behaviors, two features are prominent. **Temporal** features include the speed with which behaviors begin after stimulation (latency), how rapidly they escalate (rise time), how long they last (duration), and how slowly they go away (decay). **Intensive** features include how sensitive behaviors are to stimulation (threshold) and how strongly they express themselves (amplitude). Think what a baby's response might be to a vaccination inculcation to the arm or thigh. Temporal features of the response would be how quickly the infant begins to cry after the jab and how long the infant cries. Intensive features would be where and how long the jab was to elicit a cry and how loud the cry is. Infant temperament is inferred from these kinds of structural features of observable behaviors.

On the principle of transaction (Chapter 1), infants' individually distinctive and stable temperaments affect their current interactions and future development. Developmental scientists have uncovered many reciprocal influences between infant temperament and infants' experiences or environment. Infants' temperaments color their social interactions, their cognitions and interpretations of events, and anticipate behavioral development, among other things. For example, sociable infants tend to elicit interest and play from adults, and in turn adult social stimulation benefits infants' future development. Moreover, as infants age their temperaments lead them to prefer certain people, activities, and environments over others (especially those that best suit their individual behavioral style). For example, high-activity children might choose to pursue high-activity soccer, whereas low-activity children might opt for low-activity reading. Also, infants with different temperaments might not only shape their environments differently, but also experience their environments differently depending on their temperament.

The **goodness-of-fit**, or match, between the child's temperament and the child's context matters a great deal to the child's current functioning and later development. A child with a low activity level, positive mood, and poor adaptability fits well in a home or school setting that makes few demands and provides many opportunities for self-direction. But such an environment is a poorer fit for a child with a high activity level, high distractibility, and unhappy mood. Thus, a child's successful adjustment depends on the interaction between the child's temperament and the demands of the setting. Goodness-of-fit has important implications for infant development. A temperamentally difficult infant is not condemned to a life of later problems if parents understand and tolerate this behavioral style and provide experiences and an environment that channel and value the child's characteristics. Likewise, a happy life is not guaranteed to a temperamentally easy child if parents ignore the infant's reasonable needs or impose excessive demands on the infant. Clearly, the sensitivity and adaptability of parents to their infant's temperament is an important predictor of long-term child adjustment.

Parents and other infant caregivers devote considerable energy to identifying, adapting to, and channeling the temperaments of their infants, just as they try to interpret, respond to, and manage their infants' emotional states. In this respect, emotion and temperament have similar implications for adult caregivers. Temperament as expressed at any given time does not predetermine infants' futures. Rather, the development of infants with any particular temperament depends in part on the demands of the environments in which they live, the sensitivity and adaptability of their social partners, and the ways in which infants' temperament itself guides children's choice of activities and interpretation of their experiences. Temperament is an important, but certainly not an exclusive, determinant of infant development.

Some important considerations are how temperament is defined and measured, the genetic and experiential sources of infant temperament, as well as gender and cultural differences in temperament.

DIMENSIONS OF INFANT TEMPERAMENT

Infant temperament has a long history – probably cavemothers compared whose baby was smiling and whose was crying all the time and wondered why. In the 20th century, defining what infant temperament is turned into a keen competition among small groups of developmental scientists. One group came on the infant temperament scene in the 1950s and inaugurated the New York Longitudinal Study (NYLS; Klein, 2011). These developmental scientists interviewed mothers extensively about their 2- and 3-month-old babies. Based on these interviews, they then rated babies on nine

Table 5.1 The New York Longitudinal Study (NYLS) Infant Temperament
             Typology

Typology of Infants	Description				Percent of the NYLS Sample (%)
	Mood	Adaptability	Approach to New Situations	Intensity	
Easy	Positive	Adaptable	Positive	Low or moderate	40
Difficult	Negative	Irregular, slow	Withdraws	High	10
Slow-To-Warm-Up	Negative	Sluggish	Withdraws	Low to moderate	15
Average	Does not fit into the other profiles				35

different dimensions, including activity level, rhythmicity, attention
span, and quality of mood. The nine dimensions were thought to
be important indicators of individuality and thus good descriptions of infant temperamental styles. From the nine dimensions, the
investigators then created four broad temperamental profiles: Easy,
Difficult, Slow-To-Warm-Up, and Average (Table 5.1). Concretely,
unexpected encounters with friendly but unfamiliar adults are
experienced very differently by easy infants who are positive in
mood and adaptable in new situations versus difficult babies who
are negative in mood and slow to adapt or who withdraw quickly
from new situations.

Two notable features of the NYLS are its longevity and its clinical orientation. The investigators in question were clinicians (not
developmental scientists), and their ultimate goal was, not to
describe what infants did or why they did what they did, but to
portray stylistic features of emerging individuality in infants with
an eye to divining what the children's eventual development
would be. Faithful to their ultimate clinical goal, these clinial scientists followed their sample from infancy to young adulthood. As
clinicians, they looked for temperamental origins of later mental
and behavioral disorders. From the NYLS, they concluded that
early individuality of temperament can have long-term consequences, but temperament does not fully determine later development. They found that prediction from infancy is challenging and

often only moderate, but prediction from childhood to maturity is increasingly accurate. Some behavioral features of children in the NYLS proved to have strong influences on their later development. For example, high levels of aggression early in childhood predicted adjustment problems in adolescence. However, early individuality of temperament was not always predictive, in part (as we have learned) because temperament and the environment jointly determine goodness-of-fit. Fit with the environment at any one time might be good or bad, and fit also changes with development. Experience and environment can reinforce certain attributes of temperament or modify others. In consequence, temperament itself might change.

In the second half of the 20th century, with advances in understanding of genetics and clear temperamental styles in infants identified, a natural deduction was that temperament must be genetic in origin. Inevitably, a second group of developmental scientists came on the scene who viewed infant temperament as expressing inherited personality traits (Buss & Plomin, 1984). These behavioral geneticists regarded temperament as an early core of personality and so added dimensions to the prevailing typology, including, for example, motivation. They viewed temperament as having exclusively genetic origins and thought that temperament should be highly stable throughout life and exert enduring effects on personality. Rather than nine dimensions, this group identified only three that appear very early in life, are strongly inherited, and function independent of one another: activity level, negative emotionality, and sociability. In the purity of the genetics approach, the environment was deemed to have only limited effect on temperament. For example, children with high activity levels who was their rooms may, nevertheless, still manage to expend a great amount of energy in that setting.

The dominant contemporary view of infant temperament, spearheaded by U.S. psychologist Mary Rothbart (1940–), integrates developmental perspectives with work from psychobiology, classical conditioning, cognitive sciences, and adult personality (Rothbart, 2012). This third group partitions infant temperament into three higher-order domains, Extraversion/Surgency, Negative Affectivity, and Effortful Control, each with three or four subordinate facets (Table 5.2). This conceptualization also emphasizes development: Temperament can be modified over time via experience and environment and because the biological response systems in the brain that support temperament grow, mature, and change in development. Dimensions of temperament are also stable, but their

Table 5.2 The Prevailing Typology of Infant Temperament

Dimension	Extraversion/ Surgency	Negative Affectivity	Effortful Control
Facets	Positive affect	Fear	Attention-shifting and focusing
	Activity level	Anger	Perceptual sensitivity
	Impulsivity	Sadness	Inhibitory and activational control
		Discomfort	

Note: From Rothbart (2012).

stability is confined to periods of developmental constancy and not periods of developmental change; that is, the stability of temperament depends on when it is measured.

GENETICS AND EXPERIENCE SHAPE INFANT TEMPERAMENT

Unsurprisingly, developmental science has today converged on the position that the combined influences of nature and nurture shape infant temperament. Of course, different investigators have studied different influences. Biologically oriented investigators have sought to identify hereditary and constitutional factors and their links to temperament in two kinds of studies: one concerning the brain correlates of temperamental styles in children and the other concerning the heritability of differences in temperament. An example of the first is a longitudinal study (Kagan & Snidman, 2004) that classified 4-month-old infants as either high in reactivity (showing high levels of motor activity and distress in response to a battery of auditory, olfactory, and visual stimuli) or low in reactivity (showing low-level reactions to the same stimuli). In consonance with a biological view, reactivity showed two key characteristics. One was that reactivity was fairly stable over time. Children classified as highly reactive in infancy were likely to react fearfully to novel stimuli at 14 and 21 months, they showed little spontaneity and sociability with adults by 4½ years, they were likely to behave anxiously by 7 years, and they confessed to generalized social anxiety disorders in adolescence. A second key biological characteristic was a difference detected in specific brain limbic structures (the amygdala) that mediate fear and defense. High-reactive infants show fearful, wary, and shy behaviors, whereas low-reactive infants are generally more outgoing and emotionally flexible. fMRI examinations at 21 years revealed more activity in the amygdala in high-reactive adults than low-reactive adults when viewing novel, as opposed to familiar, faces.

An example of the second biologically oriented developmental science study that has sought to identify hereditary and constitutional factors and their links to temperament concerns the heritability of differences in temperament (Gagne & Goldsmith, 2011). Insights into the heritability of temperament come from twin studies and formal genetic analyses. As recalled from Chapter 1, researchers study infant twins to determine whether certain structures or functions have identifiable genetic roots. Monozygotic (MZ) twins share 100% of their genes, whereas dizygotic (DZ) twins share only 50% on average (as do siblings). If a structure or function has a significant genetic component, MZ twins ought to be more similar to each other than DZ twins because MZ twins share more genetic material than DZ twins. In general, twin studies indicate that individual differences in some facets of temperament are heritable. Correlations between MZ twins in temperament dimensions regularly exceed correlations between DZ twins. On these bases, the behavior genetics approach to temperament advocates that people are inclined by their unique genetic endowments to act and respond to experiences in particular ways, that their genetic endowments guide the selection of environmental settings and partners within settings that are consistent with their heritable behavioral style, and that temperament affects the environment because it evokes reactions that are consistent with genotypic characteristics. Further advances in genetic analyses have revealed that reactivity is governed by specific genes.

Reading newspaper announcements about sexy discoveries in genetics predisposes people to believe too readily that early genetic influences have immutable and unchanging consequences. However, it is wise to remember that behavioral geneticists themselves do not believe this judgment for several reasons. First, heritability estimates are specific to the population being studied, and the heritability of certain dispositional attributes are likely different in different populations; that is, heritability is not 100%, and the degree to which one or another trait is heritable varies with the group of people being studied. Second, gene action itself varies over time. Third, genetics may be inconsistent, and heredity programming changes over time. Finally, experiences can alter temperament by modifying the biological systems through which genes affect behavior.

Experientially minded developmental scientists also have their say about the origins and development of infant temperament.

Very early in life, parents assist in the development of reactivity by engaging their infant's attention. By showing their infants new objects, encouraging their infants' exploration of new people and environments, and/or by reading to their infants parents engage and change systems that underlie attention and regulation. Parents who make concerted efforts to modify their children's attributes can do so successfully. For example, intervention programs exist that successfully teach parents to help their 3- to 5-year-old children who are at risk for social anxiety disorders to be less anxious.

INFANT TEMPERAMENT AND THE WHOLE-CHILD VIEW

Individuality of temperament affects cognitive processing in infancy, and cognitive processing affects temperament. On the one hand, certain attributes of temperament might facilitate cognitive and verbal performance directly. Infants who enjoy a positive affect and are persistent in duration of orienting likely approach cognitive tasks more constructively than infants who are negative or distractible. Babies who are congenitally distractible are likely to learn slowly about objects they see because they do not attend to or concentrate on them for long periods. Five-month-olds who score high in focused attention, a dimension of temperament related to orienting, have larger vocabularies at 20 months of age (Dixon & Smith, 2008). Temperament might also affect infants' cognitive functioning indirectly by evoking certain responses from others. If parents interact more positively with infants who have positive and persistent temperaments, these characteristics could indirectly foster infants' mental development because the social responses they promote enhance development. In addition, infants with positive temperament characteristics may receive better scores on measures of cognitive performance because they respond better to unfamiliar examiners, adapt better to unfamiliar testing procedures, and/or are perceived more positively by testers.

INFANT TEMPERAMENT, GENDER, AND CULTURE

Two other questions about infant temperament are asked regularly by parents and developmental scientists. Are boys and girls alike in their temperaments? And what about infants from different cultures? Science is both cumulative and self-correcting, meaning that successive generations of developmental scientists consistently contribute to the literature in a specific area and their findings allow the field to accept replicable findings and jettison chaff. The result is the confirmation of convergent aggregate findings from increasingly larger numbers of studies. Doing so in science is called meta-analysis. A meta-analysis of the results of numerous studies of temperament involving children aged 3 months to 13 years reported that girls are rated higher in one dimension of temperament (effortful control) and boys rated higher in another (extraversion/surgency; Else-Quest et al., 2006). There was no difference between boys and girls on negative affectivity. However, not all studies find gender differences in the first year, raising questions about when and how consistent gender differences might emerge.

When cultural groups are compared, culture and gene pool are naturally **confounded**, so it is difficult to determine whether any identifiable differences in temperament are due to differences in cultural customs and socialization practices or to genetic differences between populations. This confound is one reason why researchers have focused on cultural differences in neonates or very young infants, presumably well before cultural customs or socialization practices could take hold. One study compared temperament in infants between 3 and 12 months in the United States, Poland, Russia, and Japan and found differing rates of positive and negative behaviors (Gartstein et al., 2010). Polish infants received the highest scores for Extraversion/Surgency (Positive affectivity), Japanese and Russian infants showed the highest levels of Negative Affectivity (fear). Differences in temperament might be attributable to differences in cultural ideology which, in turn, affect parenting practices. For example, in Japan and Russia infants spend little time away from their mothers and as a result may show more fear under unusual circumstances than infants from Poland or the United States where infants are away from working mothers for long periods.

SELF

Infants emote in response to people and experiences, and infants have distinct temperaments. Both emotions and temperament are outward facing, in the sense that emotions and temperament display infants' feelings to others. Infants themselves also feel, and they do so out of a rapidly developing sense of self. When and how do infants become self-aware, that is know themselves as distinct (and perhaps unique) in the world? In addition to understanding that they affect others, infants also come to understand that they are separate from others.

There are many facets to the self – a self-concept, self-esteem, self-awareness, self-identity, self-image, self-evaluation, etc. When thinking about infants, we can and cannot know certain things about infants' developing sense of self. The "self" has a venerable and layered philosophy of meanings, such as in answers to existential questions like *Who am I?*, *Where do I belong?*, and *How do I fit in?* Obviously, such questions fall well outside the bounds of infancy. But infancy harbors the glimmerings of a **self-concept**, that is an answer to the assertion *That I am*. Developing a self-concept (and later a self) is bound up with feelings of emotions and temperament, the topics of the first two sections of this chapter, and most definitely anticipate relating to others, the next chapter in this *Basics* book. In the whole-child perspective, the emergence of a self-concept depends on a brain, on perceiving, on thinking, and on relating. Indeed, many scholars believe that we develop our selves literally as social constructions and that we develop ideas about our selves strictly through processes like social comparison with others.

The self occupies a very high status in psychology. Self-awareness is central to the human experience. James, the philosopher, distinguished between the self as the knower ("I") and the self as the object that is known ("me"), and he opined that we develop a self through social interaction as we come to see ourselves as others see us. By contrast, a self-concept is the product of interior activity. Eventually, our self-concept is a view we have of our self as a physical, social, and moral being. Each of us has a self-concept, a set of ideas of who we are, and we normally think of our self as relatively constant over time. So, we come to possess an impressive degree of self-awareness that allows us to identify our self as distinct from others and to think critically about what makes us (our self) unique, including our personality, beliefs and attitudes, and likes and dislikes (even about ourselves). All this, of course, follows from infants first coming to know *that* they exist, that is achieving an understanding of themselves as individual entities with distinct characteristics.

How do we know when someone knows that they have a self? The self is private, making this question (like questions about perception and language comprehension) very tough to answer, especially before a person can talk and even speak intelligently about themselves. A traditional measure of the development of a **sense of self** is recognition of oneself in a mirror or a photograph. The mirror test, commonly referred to as the **Rouge Test**, involves surreptitiously placing a visual mark on the infant's face, usually the nose or forehead with a harmless substance like rouge, and then watching the infant's reaction when looking at her or his reflection in the mirror (Lewis, 2015). The infant's reaching for the mark (without previous training) is typically taken by developmental scientists as indicating self-awareness on the argument that this self-directed response would be impossible without a schema of one's own body (and mapping the mirror reflection onto one's own body). Infants pass the rouge test around 18 months of age. (Of course, not reaching for the rouge mark, like not expressing a preference in perception, does not indicate that the infant does not know the mark is on their body.)

A great variety of animals (from fish to chimps) has been subjected to the rouge test, and ethologists have learned that it is misconceived to construe success as a binary "Big Bang" – either you have a sense of self, or you do not. It turns out that across animal species self-awareness is gradual, as described in Box 5.2.

BOX 5.2   The Development of Self-Awareness

Just as in evolution, self-awareness passes a series of milestones as development in infancy proceeds, and each achievement builds on the previous one, layer upon layer like an onion, rather than appearing all at once like turning on a light switch.

1. First, infants are oblivious of any mirror reflection. As Piaget noted, young infants' attention focuses chiefly on the external world rather than on the self.
2. Next, infants become aware of the uniqueness of the mirror experience, especially in the perfect contingency between their own movements that are felt and seen in the mirror. This achievement indicates first glimmerings of differentiating the self from the external world. Infants display similar reactions to shadows. Likewise, other experiences give evidence that infants differentiate themselves and the world. Just as we cannot tickle ourselves, infants root to an external touch to their cheek but not to self-stimulation. To differentiate self versus other touches, infants must have some understanding of their own bodies as distinguished from others. The fact that infants imitate and that they systematically reach for objects they see, deliberately bringing their hands in contact with objects and even adjusting their grasp to unique contours of objects (Chapter 3), constitute similar evidence of self-other perceptions. That is, infants must have some (unconscious?) understanding of their bodies in relation to, but yet as separate from, other objects.
3. Finally, infants manifest self-recognition, that the image in the mirror is James's "me" and not another individual staring at and shadowing the self. Infants display this sense of self around 18 months, typically touching the mark (or rouge) and/or averting their eyes from their reflection.

How are these milestones of a self achieved? By the transacting forces of nature and nurture, of course. On the one hand, infants' neural, perceptual, and cognitive advances underpin their self-recognition in the mirror. For example, neuroimaging studies have clearly identified a brain region (specifically, the medial prefrontal cortex) that is activated in tasks that involve the self (Frewen et al., 2020). Because of age-related structural changes in this brain region, self-referential processing also changes with age. On the other hand, self-awareness is co-constructed through interactions with others (beside the obvious and trivial fact that someone has to place an infant in front of a mirror in the first place). Developmental scientists argue that self-concepts are formed in a "looking glass," that is by experiences with significant others. The character of the infant's attachment to a caregiver (a topic we explore next in Chapter 6 on Relating) leads to the construction of an **internal working model** of the self, that is the infant's representation that the self is (or is not) valuable and deserving of love and care from close others. The quality of early parenting in warmth and parental support influences the character of self-esteem at least into adulthood. Data from a nationally representative sample of 3,000 adults, ages 25–74, from the U.S. National Survey of Midlife Development concluded that parental emotional support during early childhood was a principal factor associated with decreased levels of depressive symptoms and decreased levels of chronic illness well into people's 70s (Shaw et al., 2004).

Additionally, cultures differ in how they make sense of what it means to be an individual, which aspects of the human experience are central to the self, and the resolutions to basic human dilemmas that they endorse or value. Self-concepts created in different cultural milieus adopt culture-specific ways of being, thinking, and behaving. For example, the individualist versus collectivist distinction constitutes a central organizing framework for understanding cultural differences in family life. Individualism is characterized by self-reliance, self-sufficiency, and independence, whereas collectivism is characterized by the subordination of self-oriented individual goals for the good of the group, integration, and interdependence. Exploration, autonomy, willingness to express emotion, and a positive self-concept are fostered by individualist-minded parents in the United States (for example) as opposed to dependence, emotional restraint, self-effacement, and indirect expressions of feelings as fostered by collectivist-minded parents in Japan (for example).

The significance of achieving selfhood should not be underestimated. In the whole-child view, it is noteworthy that achieving multiple more advanced developmental milestones builds on rudimentary self-awareness. A sense of self-efficacy impels the infant to explore the world, in turn stimulating cognitive, linguistic, and symbolic competencies. Only children who possess a concept of themselves as a distinct physical entity use self-referential terms (like their name or personal pronouns) and apply descriptive and evaluative terms to themselves. The secondary self-conscious emotions mentioned earlier, like embarrassment, shame, and pride, emerge and could only occur in a person who has a sense of self and is able to compare themselves with a standard. Self-evaluative emotions (being upset when caught rule breaking) and the beginnings of self-regulation (behavioral inhibition) depend on a sense of self.

To subjectively experience some level of self-esteem, children must develop a self-concept, that is a mental representation that includes at least basic beliefs about who they are physically, psychologically, and socially. As young children develop a self-concept, they form beliefs about their abilities, talents, and characteristics in different domains of life (appearance, academics, sports). Personality includes emotions and temperament but also reference to multiple aspects of the self. A permanent self-concept is a potent social force in life that influences what the child, teen, youth, or adult perceives, feels, and reacts to as well as the behaviors, perceptions, and reactions of others to that self.

SUMMARY

The infant's emotional life is complex and multidimensional. Emotional development involves changes internal to infants and changes in the behavior of infants' caregivers. With subsequent growth in a variety of developmental domains, infants' emotional repertoires broaden. Current conceptions cast temperament as a biological, early emerging, relatively stable attribute of the infant that anticipates in some degree the personality of the child. Infant temperament is conceived to be a recurring recognizable characteristic, but the consequences of temperament for later behavioral functioning are complex and not fixed. Both emotions and temperament in some sense anticipate the sense of self which dawns slowly but inevitably over the course of infancy (and well into childhood). Newborns seem not to have a sense of self, but remarkably in the space of a short year and one-half infants come to recognize that they exist as separate entities in the world. As such, they have moved from a state of *fetus ex utero*, almost autistic in their basic nature, to forceful willful interactive beings making their own demands and wishes abundantly clear ... and hardly deniable.

6

RELATING

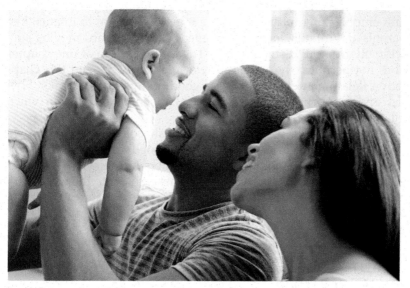

(Image courtesy of Shutterstock, copyright: Monkey Business Images/ Shutterstock.com.)

INTRODUCTION

In **Bioecological Systems Theory**, which we introduced in Chapter 1, the infant sits at the center of five nested systems that influence development (Figure 1.3; Wachs, 2015). The *microsystem* is

DOI: 10.4324/9781003172802-6

most proximal to the infant and encompasses interpersonal relationships and patterns of activities that the infant experiences in face-to-face settings. This system includes family members, daycares and schools, peers, the wider neighborhood, and material things in the infant's immediate environment. Further distant from the infant, which the infant may not directly encounter but still indirectly influence infant development, are elements of the *exosystem* like the parent's workplace and the health care system. The *macrosystem* is the most distant from the infant and encompasses patterns of beliefs, values, laws, social class, and culture where the infant grows up. Finally, as development literally implies, at any given moment the infant exists at a particular time as well as at some fixed period in history; the time domain in development is called the *chronosystem*. As ordered, these systems stand in increasingly distant relations to the infant, but each distal system influences infant development through more proximal systems.

This chapter is organized and illustrated following these systems, first emphasizing influences that are most proximal to infants, like parents and infants' local environment, and afterward moving successively to more distal systems. The limited space of one chapter does not permit coverage of all relevant influences, but this chapter on Relating attempts to offer a good understanding of just how rich and supportive to development are the many contexts in which infants are enveloped.

Before turning to describe these several ecologies of infancy, we show that infants bring many sophisticated capacities to establishing relationships with significant others in their lives (in other words, the "bio" in bioecological). Infants arrive into the world prepared to be social partners, and the people infants come into contact with in their first years of life are eager to support mutual social interactions with them.

INFANTS ARE PREPARED TO BE SOCIAL PARTNERS

People have specific bodily features, make specific sounds, emit specific odors, and move in specific ways. As recounted in earlier chapters in this *Basics* book, infants enjoy several predispositions and many abilities that help them distinguish and recognize specific people by their specific faces, voices, smells, and movements. For example, newborns prefer face-like stimuli from birth, and they look more at faces that look directly back at them – like parents do – and they remember those faces better than the same faces that avert their eye gaze. Fetuses hear *in utero*, and after birth babies look at things they hear. So, information specifying a parent's face and voice is quickly coordinated. For example, 3-month-olds match emotional sounds to emotional visual displays (laughing sounds with smiling faces) more successfully when the sounds and faces are their mother's. In turn, familiarity with their mother's voice feeds into early language acquisition. Infants attend longer to spoken passages made up of target words that they previously heard their mothers speak than words spoken by an unfamiliar stranger.

Infants quickly learn to recognize people by their smell, and breastfeeding infants recognize and prefer their mother's odor within a few days of birth. By 3 months, infants distinguish between movement patterns that specify animate versus inanimate entities, and by 5 months infants perceive the human form based on the barest of information such as presented in point-light displays.

Furthermore, infants' increasingly sophisticated cognitive abilities set them on a path to relate to others. Infants not only learn about appropriate emotions and the people who display them, they also learn about prosocial versus antisocial behaviors. In the infant world, a prosocial behavior might be helping someone up a hill, whereas an antisocial behavior might be hindering someone's progress up a hill by pushing them back or giving or taking a toy. Three-month-olds watch video enactments of helpers longer than hinderers, and between 6 and 10 months of age they prefer to interact with helpers (Hamlin, 2015). By 9 months infants can predict others' actions, and by 16 months infants discriminate accidental versus intentional actions and recognize that a hindering action could be an accident or that a helping action might fail (van de Vondervoort & Hamlin, 2018).

In short order, then, their perceptual and cognitive abilities incline infants to know things about the important people in their lives. And infants use these abilities to forge meaningful relationships. Significantly, infants do not grow up in isolation: Not only are humans of all ages intensely social creatures, human infants are **altricial**, a term from zoology (the study of the animal kingdom) that means species that are helpless at birth. Human infants cannot and do not survive on their. They but need caregivers. Indeed, British psychoanalyst D. W. Winnicott (1896–1971) quipped enigmatically, *there is no such thing as an infant*, meaning infants cannot exist, survive, or thrive without competent caregivers who nourish them, regulate their temperature, teach them, and prepare them for their future life. Interpersonal Acceptance-Rejection Theory (Rohner & Lansford, 2017) posits that human beings have developed an enduring, universal, emotional need for positive responses from the people closest to them, especially parents. If children experience parental rejection, they are likely to suffer numerous adverse physical and mental health outcomes into maturity.

Understanding infancy completely and accurately depends on appreciating the multiple significant others and social contexts in which infants develop, that is the ecologies of development we referred to at the outset of this chapter. Different contexts provide infants with different experiences that together shape infant development and prepare infants to survive and thrive in the very environments they are likely to encounter as they grow. The most proximal ecology to infants (microsystem) is created by parents, and the next part of this chapter is spent on parental caregiving. Afterward, others in the infants' microsystems are discussed and then the larger social contexts in which infants are embedded, the macro- and chronosystems, are covered.

PARENTS AND PARENTING

Parents create their infant offspring biologically, of course, but also psychologically because parents shape their infants' development in many direct and indirect ways. The direct ways are the more obvious. Parents directly endow their children with a genetic makeup, 50% from mother and 50% from father, that contributes to their infants' psychological make-up. Mothers and fathers are also responsible for virtually all of their infants' social and material experiences. In the natural course of things, these two main sorts of direct effects are **confounded**: The same parents who endow their infants with their genetics also interact socially with their infants and outfit their infants' material world. For a variety of reasons, it is desirable to identify the distinct contributions of heritable from experiential influences on infancy and infant development. One theoretical and already very familiar reason is that heritable and experiential influences harken back to the nature-nurture question. A perhaps more immediately relevant reason is that, once a child is imbued with a genetic endowment, the child's biological composition cannot normally or easily be changed. By contrast, if experience and environment matter to infant development, then the course and outcome of an infant's future can be altered, and presumably improved, by manipulating the infant's experiences and environment. Disentangling the contributions of heritable from experiential influences on infancy and infant development is difficult to do, but not impossible. So-called **natural experiments** can distinguish the part each plays.

DIRECT EFFECTS – HERITABILITY

Mothers and fathers directly contribute to their infants' nature by passing on their genes, and behavior geneticists have worked out several ways to assess the contributions of genetics and experience to many individual infant characteristics, such as physical growth, intelligence, and personality. Two main research paradigms involve twins and adoptees (as already described in Chapter 1). If a characteristic is inherited, MZ twins, even if reared apart, should be alike on the characteristic, just as MZ twins should be more alike than DZ twins. The other research paradigm examines the degree to which adopted children share traits with their adoptive versus biological parents. If a characteristic is inherited, adopted children should be more like their biological parents with whom they share genes, but not the same environment, than their adoptive parents with whom they share an environment, but not genes. If a characteristic depends on experience, then adopted children should be more like their adoptive parents with whom they share experiences, but not genes, than their biological parents with whom they share genes, but not experiences.

Using these two research strategies, behavioral geneticists have reported high degrees of heritability for a surprising range of individual characteristics as, for example, infant measures indicative of information processing, language ability, and temperament (Benson et al., 1993). Analyses of biological versus adoptive children in the same family reveal that prenatal depression in mothers affects their biological children's risk of depression via genetic pathways, but prenatal maternal drug use affects their adoptive children's risk of depression via experiential pathways. Clearly, parents significantly influence their infants' development through their own biological characteristics. However, parents (and others in the infant's life) also shape infant development by providing direct formative experiences.

DIRECT EFFECTS – PARENTING

The fact that infants inherit some characteristics does not negate or even diminish the significance of direct (and, as we show later, indirect) effects of parenting on infants. Genes might make siblings alike, but as we all know siblings are still very different. Even within the same family, parents create different experiences and environments for different children (called **nonshared environments**), and siblings' different experiences contribute in telling ways to make them distinctive individuals. Equally central to understanding infancy, therefore, is understanding the direct effects of parenting.

Developmental scientists have distinguished major domains of the experiences parents provide infants. **Nurturant caregiving** promotes infants' basic survival (protection, supervision, safety, and sustenance); **physical caregiving** fosters infants' fine and gross motor development; **social caregiving** comprises parents' efforts to engage infants in interpersonal exchanges (soothing, touching, smiling, and vocalizing); **didactic caregiving** pertains to how parents facilitate infants' understanding of the world around them (naming, labeling, directing attention to and interpreting external events, and providing opportunities to learn); and **material caregiving** involves parents outfitting and structuring infants' physical environments (visual and audio stimulation and other implements). For example, developmental scientists have studied contributors to language development in infancy by analyzing maternal language input to children as well as the richness of the infant's environment (Bornstein 2019). Mothers who speak more to their infants and are more responsive to their infants (social and didactic caregiving) have infants who later command more language, and mothers who outfit their infants' environment with books and pictures and who change wall-hangings regularly (material caregiving) also have infants who later have more language. Notable is that each parenting domain makes independent contributions to infants' language.

These parenting domains seem to operate according to several known tenets. One is the specificity principle, which states that specific domains of parenting at specific times shape specific infant abilities in specific ways. For example, mothers' verbal responsiveness to infants' vocalizations at around 1 year (how prompt, appropriate, and contingent mothers are verbally to their infants when their infants vocalize) predicts infants' later language, but not their play competence, at around 2 years. By contrast, mothers' responsiveness to their infants' play at around 1 year predicts the sophistication of infant play, not language, at around 2 years (Tamis-LeMonda & Bornstein, 1994). A second tenet of parent–infant relationships (introduced in Chapter 1) is the transaction principle, which states that infants shape their experiences with parents just as they are shaped by those experiences. Interactions between parents and infants emulate an intricate dance in rhythm and in style. Who leads and who follows is often not clear. So, infants are influenced by their environment, but they also alter their environment as they interact with it, and they interpret the environment in their own ways. In shorter words, infant and environment actively shape one another through time. For example, the extent to which infants are perceived as easy or difficult in their temperament may influence how parents respond to them, and the quality of parents' response, in turn, further shapes infant development (Bridgett et al., 2009, 2018). A third tenet of parenting is domain independence, which refers to the fact that the different modes of caregiving are largely unrelated to one another. For example, mothers who engage in social interactions with their infants more are not necessarily or automatically more or less didactic with their infants. Fourth, although parenting domains are conceptually separate, they still can (and do) occur simultaneously as, for example, when a mother reads to her infant (didactic caregiving) by placing the infant on her lap and caressing her child at the same time (social caregiving).

Finally, these parenting domains have developmental dimensions. Recall from Box 1.3 that **stability** is consistency in the relative positions of individuals in a group over time, and **continuity** is consistency in the mean level of group performance over time. A substantial amount of longitudinal developmental science has shown that direct experiences parents provide are fairly consistent during their children's early years. For example, some mothers talk a lot to their infants, whereas other mothers do so less. Mothers who are prone to talk a lot to their 2-month-olds are likely to talk a lot when their infants are 24-month-olds. Stability of such individual differences is different from group-level continuity. Parenting can be expected to change as children develop from neonate to infant to toddler: As a group, parents talk more to their 2-year-olds than to their 2-month-olds. Also, around the middle of the first year, the nature of infant–mother interaction changes from almost exclusively social to combinations of social and didactic. That is, caregiving is not static, but constantly changing to keep apace of infant development. Parents' direct influences on infants consist of their genetic endowment as well as their actual parenting cognitions and practices.

MOTHERS AND FATHERS

Because mothers have traditionally assumed primary, if not exclusive, responsibility for infant care, theorists and researchers interested in infancy have been much more concerned with mothering than fathering of infants. And even though society has witnessed increasing interest in childrearing on the part of fathers, to this day mothers still bear the largest responsibility for infants and most societies place stronger emphases (and burdens) on the

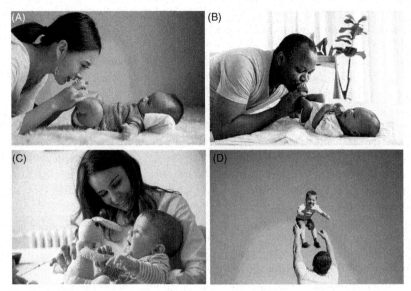

Figure 6.1 Similarities in mothers (A) and fathers (B), and differences between mothers (C) and fathers (D) in caring for their young infants. (Image courtesy of Shutterstock, copyright: nokkaew/ Shutterstock.com, Anatta_Tan/Shutterstock.com, BalanceForm Creative/Shutterstock.com, Guas/Shutterstock.com.)

mother–infant relationship. Close investigation has revealed that mothers and fathers interact with and care for their infants in ways that are both strikingly similar (Figure 6.1A and B) and remarkably different (Figure 6.1C and D). In terms of some similarities, when observed feeding their infants, both fathers and mothers respond to their infants' cues either with social bids or by adjusting the pace of the feeding, and mothers' language and fathers' language to infants both promote children's language development. In terms of differences, fathers around the world typically spend less time with their infants than mothers, and fathers typically see themselves (as they are seen by their partners and others) as helpers rather than the parent with primary responsibility for infant caregiving. Mothers and fathers also tend to engage infants in contrasting activities: In face-to-face play with their 3-week- to 6-month-old infants, for example, fathers tend to engage infants in staccato bursts of physical and social stimulation, whereas mothers tend to be more rhythmic and hold infants more. Overall, mothers are prone to nurture infants and fathers to play with them.

INDIRECT EFFECTS

Parents influence infants through interactions they have with them – direct effects – but also by how parents influence one another – indirect effects. For example, some paternal influences on infant development are indirectly mediated through fathers' impact on mothers and vice versa. Fathers who are emotionally supportive of mothers, share household chores, maintain a harmonious and contented mood in the household, and provide for family material needs reduce stresses on mothers and so improve the qualities of mothering and mother–infant relationships (Parke & Cookston, 2019). Conversely, mothers often control the extent to which fathers are involved with the children, called **maternal gatekeeping** (Lee et al., 2019).

DETERMINANTS OF PARENTING INFANTS

Infants do not come with an operating manual. How do parents know what to do? Developmental scientists concede that the origins of parenting are extremely complex. One parenting researcher identified more than 30 factors that affect parenting, and that was more than a quarter-century ago, before parenting research really blossomed. Here, we briefly discuss five general spheres of influence thought to be to be especially important in understanding the determinants of parenting.

1. *Parents' Own Characteristics.* Several biological and psychological characteristics of parents shape their parenting. On the biological side, both maternal and paternal hormones change during pregnancy, as do mothers' and fathers' brains, in ways that influence their parenting (see Chapter 2). An example hormone is oxytocin, which increases during pregnancy and promotes sociality and face recognition (Peltola et al., 2018). Parenting is also affected by parent age. The average age of mothers at first birth in the United States is currently around 26 years, but adolescent parenthood is still common (perhaps 1 in 3 U.S. adolescent women becomes pregnant by the end of her 19th year) and more and more women in their 30s and 40s are giving birth today. Infants born to younger and older parents are at greater biological and social risks. For example, teenage and older mothers tend to report higher levels of parenting stress compared to mothers in their 20s and early 30s. On the psychological side, parenting reflects adult personality traits as does the state of parents' mental health (Bornstein,

2016). Psychologically open parents respond to infants in one way, but neurotic parents in a different way; depressed or alcoholic parents behave toward infants differently from mentally healthy parents. Later this chapter describes attachment relationships between parents and infants. Mothers' attachment relationships with their own parents impact the way they interact with their own infants (Sroufe, 2017).

2.   *Parents' Cognitions.* Parents hold informal theories of child development, such as what behaviors are appropriate for what ages, and parents continually assess their infants' level of development when deciding how best and most productively to interact with them. In addition, perceived efficacy as a parent affects parents' sensitivity because parents who feel effective are motivated to engage their infants in interaction, which in turn provides additional opportunities to read their infants' signals, interpret them, and respond to them. Finally, parents who believe that they have little or no effect on their infant's intelligence or temperament are unlikely to take active roles in their infants' development.

3.   *Situational Influences.* Situations in which parents find themselves with infants (the bath versus supermarket checkout line), tasks parents must accomplish (feeding, getting the baby to sleep), and immediate demands on parents (working, answering the phone) as well as family structure (having one infant or several children) and family systems (being a single parent or cohabiting), support networks that surround parents (availability of childcare), employment obligations (full-time homemaker or full-time employment outside the home), and the neighborhoods where they live (safe and secure or dangerous and chaotic) all shape the parenting of infants and affect parents' attentiveness, patience, stress, and tolerance.

4.   *Parents' Social Class, Ethnicity, and Culture.* This chapter concludes with an expanded look at each of these larger contextual forces that shape parenting and, via parenting, influence infancy.

5.   *Actual or Perceived Infant Characteristics.* Infants differ in their temperaments, so one parenting practice that rapidly soothes one infant may be ineffective with another infant. Thus, parents of different infants may reach different conclusions about their parenting practices or their own competence as parents. Infants differ in responsiveness (the extent and quality of their reactivity to stimulation), readability (the definitiveness

of their behavioral signals), and predictability (the degree to which their behaviors can be anticipated reliably from their own preceding behaviors or contextual events). The health and developmental maturity of infants also affect parents and the quality of parenting, as has been illustrated in research on preterm infants and infants later identified as having ASD or any myriad diseases (from ear infections to cancer). For example, mothers of preterm infants are more active and directive in their parenting than are mothers of term infants (Gattis, 2019).

It is seductive, but useless, to ask whether one or another of these spheres of influence is more important than the others. Each determinant plays a part in the origins and expression of what parents think and how they act. In addition, all of these factors co-occur. That is, every person who becomes a parent has a biology and a psychology, a social class, ethnicity, and culture. It is challenging in the extreme to unpackage the impacts these factors have, separately or together.

ATTACHMENT

Practically speaking, infants' capabilities and parents' practices serve many functions and are geared to achieve many goals, not the least important of which is the attachment between infant and caregiver. **Attachments** are specific, enduring, emotional bonds between people, and they are of major importance in infancy and the social and mental development of children. Bowlby (1969) originated the notion of attachment based on observations of WWII orphans. Because of its significance, we first recount developmental stages of infant attachment which Bowlby described, then the measurement of attachment, and the classifications of attachment that fall out of its measurement. Next, we focus on behavior systems that underpin infant attachment and sources of variations in attachment. We conclude with accounts of the stability and predictive validity of attachment classifications.

STAGES OF ATTACHMENT DEVELOPMENT

Bowlby (1969) described three important phases in the development of infant–parent attachments and their approximate ages: (1) a phase of indiscriminate social responsiveness that lasts from birth to 2 months, (2) a phase of discriminating sociability that lasts from 2 to 7 months, and (3) full-blown attachment beginning at 7 months.

From birth, babies cry, which of course motivates adults to pick them up and soothe them by talking, caressing, and/or nourishing. Around the second month of life, babies begin to smile, which like crying, powerfully shapes adult behavior (Figure 5.1). These examples demonstrate that infants are capable of affecting the social environment around them, and adults respond to infants' behaviors and signals. Cries encourage adults to approach a baby, and smiles encourage adults to stay near a baby. Crying and smiling are infants' first-emerging attachment behaviors. Both cues bring the baby into close protective comfort and security with a caregiving adult, but any adult will do. In this sense, in the first 2 months of life infants interact with people but prefer no particular person; they are **indiscriminately sociable**. Other caregiving routines, including feeding and social play, provide other contexts for social interaction, and because infants' caregivers can be seen, heard, smelled, and felt, babies come to learn about them in particular.

On the basis their budding attention to and memory for specific faces and experiences with specific people, and because certain people have come to be associated with pleasurable experiences (e.g., feeding, cuddling, rocking, and play) as well as relief of distress (due, say, to hunger), babies come to prefer to interact with those familiar people. Around 2 months, infants adopt a **discriminating sociability** for certain people (typically their parents) over others. Those certain people are able to soothe the baby more easily and elicit smiles and babbles more readily and regularly. (Recall how the still-face procedure disrupts infants' expectations for these interactions; Chapter 4). During this second phase of social development, infants' distress diminishes, they are more behaviorally coordinated, their arousal levels become less variable, and they spend longer periods of time in an alert state. Reciprocally at about this time, parents come to enjoy being special to their baby and are enormously rewarded by positive displays in their baby's behavior. By the end of this phase, at about 7 months, specific attachments emerge.

During the second half of the first year, infants also learn that what they do can affect what others do in return; developmental scientists have termed this ability of infants **effectance**. Infants also learn **trust**, or the expectation that a particular caregiver can be counted on to respond quickly and appropriately when signaled. These lessons constitute significant milestones on the way to becoming social. In such relationships, infants learn that their cries, smiles, and babbles elicit predictable responses from others and so infants gain confidence in their predictions that others will respond to them. Developing a sense of trust and effectance leads to the third phase of attachment.

By about 7 months of age, infants are beginning to prefer interacting with certain people or **attachment figures**. At around this time, infants are also crawling, and therefore can get close to their caregivers instead of waiting for caregivers to respond to their cries, smiles, or babbles. Infants are increasingly likely to initiate interactions, assuming increasingly active roles in their interpersonal relationships. And they balance keeping in physical proximity to caregivers and exploring their environment. For their part, attachment figures provide a **secure base** from which infants explore.

One example of effectance is infants protesting (often by crying) when attachment figures depart. Separation protests aim at making attachment figures return. From about 7 to 24 months, infants become increasingly sophisticated in their abilities to behave intentionally and communicate verbally. They tolerate growing distances from attachment figures, and they also become more and more adept at interacting with unfamiliar adults. Box 6.1 describes other main features of attachment.

BOX 6.1 Main Features of Attachment

1. Infants become attached to people who are consistent, predictable, and appropriate in responding to their signals and needs.
2. Over and above some minimum amount of time adults spend with infants, the quality of adult–infant interaction determines whether attachments form and what character they take.
3. Most infants form attachments to both their parents at about the same time, and infants display equivalent attachment behaviors (propensity to stay near, approach, touch, cry to, and be held) to both parents.
4. In the absence of a consistent caregiver (as might occur in institutions such as orphanages), infants do not form secure attachments.
5. Most babies develop a "hierarchy" of attachment figures, and their primary caregivers become primary attachment figures before other relationships are formed. When distressed, infants increase displays of attachment behaviors and organize their behavior similarly around whichever parent is present. When both parents are present, however, distressed infants tend to turn to mothers preferentially.
6. Once infants have the foundation of a primary attachment figure, they may form relationships with others, for example, fathers, grandparents, older siblings, and daycare workers.

Clearly, and in accord with the whole-child view, perception and cognition play central roles in infants' developing attachments. **Theory of mind** is the ability to attribute mental states – beliefs, intents, desires, pretending, knowledge – to oneself and others and to understand that others have mental states that differ from one's own. Infants are deeply egocentric in this respect, and do not recognize that others' perspectives differ from their own. Piaget opined about the gradual decentration in cognition that takes place over the first years of life, and Bowlby described a fourth stage of attachment development when children come to understand that attachment figures have mental states that sometimes differ from children's own. There is an active debate in the infancy research community about when infants and children acquire a theory of mind, but it is known that children who have secure attachment relationships enjoy a more advanced understanding of others' mental states. So, positive social interactions not only build on earlier neurological, attentional, and perceptual capacities but also facilitate cognitive and socioemotional development. Acquiring a theory of mind might also depend on the development of a sense of self.

MEASUREMENT AND CLASSIFICATIONS OF INFANT–PARENT ATTACHMENTS

A student of Bowlby, Ainsworth developed a procedure – the **Strange Situation** – to assess infant attachment. This seven-episode research protocol is best used when infants are about 10 to 24 months of age – old enough to have formed attachments and to be mobile but still young enough to tolerate brief separations and encounters with strangers (Ainsworth & Wittig, 1969). Episodes usually last 3 minutes but can be extended or abbreviated if the infant becomes distressed. At base the procedure exposes infants to increasing amounts of stress to observe how they organize their attachment behaviors around their parents. An unfamiliar environment, the entrance of an unfamiliar adult, and two brief separations from the parent induce stress.

At the beginning of the procedure, the infant and parent enter a playroom. The infant should use a parent attachment figure as a secure base from which to explore the novel environment. A stranger's entrance should lead the infant to inhibit exploration and draw closer to the parent. The parent's departure should lead the infant to attempt to bring the parent back by crying or searching, and their exploration and affiliation with the stranger reduce. Following the parent's return, the infant should seek to re-engage the parent in interaction, and, if distressed, the infant may wish to be cuddled and comforted. The same responses should occur, with somewhat greater intensity, following a second separation and reunion.

The majority of infants, about 60% in the United States, behave as just described, which according to Ainsworth is the optimal way babies should behave in relation to their attachment figure. These infants are said to have a **secure attachment.** Some 10–15% of infants in U.S. samples are unable to use their parents as secure bases to explore, and although they are distressed by their parents' departure they behave ambivalently on reunion: They seek contact and also angrily reject the parent. These infants are conventionally described as having an **insecure-resistant attachment.** A third group of about 20% of the infants in U.S. samples gives the impression that they are unconcerned by their parent's absence, and instead of greeting the parent on reunion, they actively avoid interaction and ignore their parent's bids for reunion. These infants are said to exhibit **insecure-avoidant attachments.** Finally, about 5–10% of infants in U.S. samples simultaneously display contradictory behavior patterns, make incomplete movements, and appear confused or apprehensive about approaching their parent. These infants are classified as having a **disorganized attachment.**

Secure attachments enjoy open, flexible communication between parents and their children around emotion signals and balance a range of positive and negative emotions. By contrast, insecure attachments are characterized by problematic communications of emotions, where parents and children exhibit a restricted range of emotions or heighten displays of emotion. We stipulated "U.S. samples" in this account because (as discussed at the end of this chapter) infants with different cultural histories fall into the same four categories but in different proportions.

SOURCES OF INFANT–PARENT ATTACHMENT

Why are some infants securely attached and others not? The origins of individual differences in infants' behavior in the Strange Situation have been debated. At this point in this *Basics* book, it should be no surprise that some authorities attribute infant behavior in the Strange Situation to infants' experience with prior infant–parent interactions (nurture), whereas others attribute behavior in the Strange Situation to infants' temperament (nature). Also, it is no surprise that it is likely that both nature and nurture shape infant security. According to attachment theory, the quality of children's interactions with caregivers over time creates an **internal working model** of their relationships with specific people, how relationships work, and children's own value in relationships. In general, **sensitive parenting** that is nurturant, attentive, responsive, and nonrestrictive is associated with secure infant behavior in the Strange Situation. Infants who enjoy a history with attachment figures who protect them and are consistently responsive and accessible when needed develop a secure internal working model of their relationship. By contrast, infants who have learned not to trust attachment figures tend to be insecure. Insecure-resistant attachments have been linked to inconsistent, unresponsive parenting, and insecure-avoidant attachments with intrusive and over-stimulating or rejecting parenting. Disorganized attachments have been found among abused and maltreated infants and may be consequences of parental behaviors that infants find frightening or disturbing.

Insecure attachments deserve a second thought. Although they appear to be non optimal, it might be more valid to conceptualize them as adaptive responses to non optimal caregiving environments. If a parent is not consistently responsive to the infant's needs, for example, not to rely on the parent (an insecure-avoidant attachment) might represent a good coping strategy. This line of reasoning is consistent with the **Adaptive Calibration Model** that posits that individual differences develop as adaptations to meet the conditions of current or future environments (Del Giudice et al., 2011).

Developmental scientists tend to point to infants' interactive history as predictive of their attachment classification, but infant temperament (which we learned in Chapter 5 has a biological basis) might affect infants' security of attachment via several indirect routes. One indirect effect comes about because temperament affects the quality of infant–parent interaction. For example, temperamentally attentive babies might be more affected by their parents' behavior than temperamentally distractible babies.

Thus, the quality of infant–parent interaction might determine whether a child will become securely or insecurely attached, but constitutionally based differences in temperament would determine whether the child's insecurity will be manifest in a low distress (avoidant) or high distress (resistant) manner.

BEHAVIOR SYSTEMS THAT UNDERPIN ATTACHMENT

Attachment behaviors promote proximity between infants and adults. The goal is to ensure closeness and protection with obvious adaptive value. Four systems are thought to underpin attachment. One is the **attachment behavior system**. This system controls infant activities that attain and maintain proximity to or contact with attachment figures on whom the infant can rely for nurturance and protection. Examples are crying, gestures, or other signals that indicate the desire to be comforted. Attachment behaviors are usually directed to persons with whom infants are attached. The attachment behavior system has adaptive significance in that it increases the probability of infant survival. In contrast is the **fear/wariness behavior system**, which coordinates avoidant, wary, or fearful responses to strangers. These behaviors are also adaptive in that there is survival value in avoiding unknown and potentially dangerous persons and situations. Apprehension over the appearance of strange persons emerges around 7 to 8 months of age, about the same time infants begin to prefer certain people (their attachment figures).

It may be adaptive to be wary when first encountering strangers, but it is not adaptive to avoid all interactions with nonattachment figures. Interactions with many people other than parents are vital to children's wholesome mental and social development. It is not surprising, therefore, that wariness diminishes over time, and infants eventually enter into friendly interactions with nonattachment figures. These kinds of interactions initially involve social behaviors at a distance (such as smiling and vocalizing) and are mediated by an **affiliative behavior system**. Infants also engage with their physical environment using an **exploratory behavior system** to investigate and manipulate objects that also facilitates the development of cognitive competencies.

Activation of the attachment and fear/wariness systems is incompatible with affiliation and exploration systems. So, affiliation and exploration are inhibited when either the attachment or the fear/wariness system is activated. And the reverse is also true. What does this dynamic look like in actual infant behavior we can observe? When infants are not distressed and are in familiar surroundings, they might freely engage in interaction with less familiar persons (activation of the affiliative system) and actively explore the environment (activation of the exploratory system) while remaining near their attachment figures (i.e., the fear/wariness system is either not activated or is inhibited).

STABILITY AND PREDICTIVE VALIDITY OF INFANT ATTACHMENT

Infant attachment status has taken on outsized importance because short- and long-term studies in developmental science have revealed that infant attachment status tends to be stable in the short run (attachment classification tells us something about individual infants that persists) and predictive in the long run (attachment classification tells us something about what individual infants will be like as older children). The individual's internal working model is an unconscious representation of early intimate ties primarily with caregivers, and has been theorized that, once formed, remains relatively constant over development. The notion that Strange Situation behaviors are intrinsic to infant relationships and not ephemeral is supported by some findings (but certainly not all) that attachment classifications of infants are stable over time. In one study, 96% of infants were awarded the same attachment classification at 12 and at 18 months of age (Waters, 1978); other studies have documented stability between 12-month assessments in the Strange Situation and 6-year assessments of attachment measured in other ways (Main & Cassidy, 1988). One review of the literature concluded that attachment security is at least moderately stable across the first 19 years of life (Fraley, 2002). Notably, however, material and social changes in the infant's environment are known to erode stability. For example, in a low-SES sample when families experienced social and economic stress secure attachments often changed to insecure; the birth of a second child sometimes predicts a decrease in attachment security among firstborn children. Thus, all is not set at 7 months of age (see Box 6.2).

Not insignificantly as well, attachment classifications appear to predict aspects of children's future behavior, albeit in imperfect degree. Specifically, cognitive internal working models guide feelings, behaviors, and how information about the world is processed. As well, children are believed to learn both sides of the attachment relationship. For example, secure infants compared to insecure infants learn whether significant others in their lives will come to their aid when they need help, as well as ways of responding to the distress of others. They have fewer behavior problems themselves, and they engage in more frequent, more prosocial, and more mature forms of interaction with their siblings and peers, as measured by sharing more and showing a greater capacity to initiate and maintain interactions (Sroufe, 2017). Similarly, infants with secure attachments to their mothers later play more cooperatively when interacting with a friendly stranger. In addition, secure infants at 12 or 18 months persist longer and more indefatigably on challenging cognitive tasks and display superior problem-solving abilities in stressful and challenging contexts in the preschool years than do insecure children. Insecure (especially disorganized) attachment in infancy predicts antisocial behavior, depression, and anxiety in later childhood (Groh et al., 2012). Preschoolers (children aged 3–5 years) with a history of

BOX 6.2   Set for Life? Learning to Love Again

Can children with initially insecure attachments develop secure attachments with others? The loving, attentive, responsive care that infants receive from their parents over the first months of life lead them to form trusting and loving attachment relationships. In the normal course of affairs, these relationships continue to deepen over the succeeding months and appear to form the social and emotional foundations that shape children's characteristic reactions to people as well as their responses to cognitive and emotional challenges they will confront in the years ahead. When children experience maltreatment rather than sensitive responsive care at the hands of their parents, they nevertheless form attachments to the abusive parents, although these relationships are often the disorganized type even when those children have been able to develop and maintain secure attachments to other (non abusing) parents and care providers. What happens when these infants are removed from their families and placed in foster homes? Can these infants form attachments to new parent figures, despite having spent their early, attachment-forming months in conditions that were so poor that social service agencies had to intervene?

Stovall-McClough and Dozier (2004) used detailed diary entries by foster parents to assess the status of the infants' behavior with them. The majority of fostered infants showed signs that they were developing attachments to their foster mothers within the first 2 months that they were together. Nearly 60% of the attachments also appeared to be secure, and the likelihood that these infants would develop secure rather than insecure relationships was evident from differences in their behavior in the first week or two after placement (Bernier et al., 2004). The younger the infants were when first placed with the foster families – some were as young as 5 months – the more likely they were to develop secure attachments to their foster mothers. Because secure attachments appear to offer many benefits to children, these findings strongly suggest that maltreated infants should be removed from inadequate parents and placed with foster or adoptive parents. Dozier and colleagues (2009) later showed that foster mothers can successfully be trained to interact more sensitively with their foster infants, and that foster mothers' increased sensitivity in turn facilitates infants' better adaptation to their new homes.

insecure-resistant or insecure-avoidant attachments with their caregivers tend to be victimized by peers.

From the whole-child perspective, infants' security status reflects conjoint neural, motor, perceptual, cognitive, and temperamental aspects of infant development. For example, advances in motor development over the first 2 years increase infants' opportunities to interact with people and objects. Once infants can reach, they can engage with the objects that others give them; once they are capable of self-produced locomotion, they can initiate interactions with the people around them. At this time, infants also begin to share. While exploring their world, they may turn to an adult, usually a parent, and show or give an object (Figure 6.2).

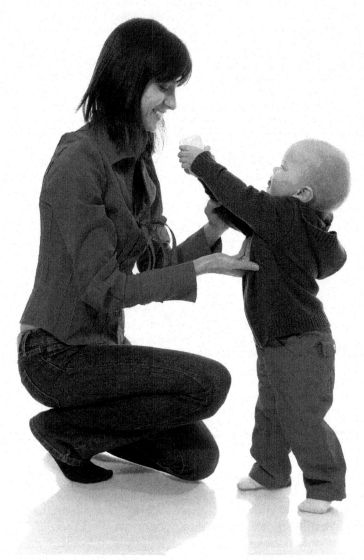

Figure 6.2 An infant sharing with mother. (Image Courtesy of Shutterstock, Inc. Copyright: Olga Sapegina/Shutterstock.com.)

INFANT GENDER

Before moving beyond the infant and the infant-parent microsystem to consider the relationships of other important people in infants' lives, we interrupt the narrative to comment briefly on the role of infant gender in relating. Infants bring many characteristics to their relationships with others, like their temperament, and gender may also be important in this regard. The infant's gender may be associated with differences in behavioral style and how the infant interprets the world, as well the ways in which others perceive and relate to the child.

Evidence about innate gender differences in children is perennially controversial. One of the very first questions parents and others ask about a newborn is what "sex" the baby is, and the phenomenon of prenatal "gender reveal parties," a practice that originated in the early 2000s, amply attests to the central importance of sex/gender in the lives of the child's family and friends-to-be. Then or very soon after, gifts, clothes, and room decorations for baby girls and boys are likely to be strictly sex stereotyped.

It turns out, however, that most differences between girl and boy infants are in the "eye of the beholder," and very few withstand objective analysis. There is some evidence that male infants are more active than female infants and that female infants show more distress or fear to novelty than male infants. But, among all the neural, motor, perceptual, cognitive, emotional, temperamental, and social possibilities, that's about it. Female and male fetuses are exposed to different hormonal environments which might account for some small gender differences in some infant behaviors. For example, females exposed to testosterone *in utero* make masculine toy choices between 3 and 10 years of age, despite the fact that parents encouraged feminine toy choices (Pasterski et al., 2005). For the vast majority of structures and functions, the individual variability among girls and among boys is respectively so wide as to swamp any meaningful differences between the two. Where once a literature on sex differences thrived, closer scrutiny on the part of developmental scientists has rejected those notions dramatically in major support of a gender similarities hypothesis. That is, commonly believed gender difference stereotypes are more apparent than real, and when researchers take a hard empirical look, most "differences" between girls and boys (outside of genitalia and reproductive systems) fall by the wayside.

Unfortunately, objective evidence-based similarities sometimes fail to supplant subjective opinions. Parents constitute initial influences on the development of their infants' gender, and parents have marked tendencies to treat children differently by gender. Classic "Baby X" studies (where the gender of the infant is not known to study participants) have revealed that parents (and other adults) conceive of and behave toward infants differently depending on whether they *think* they are interacting with a girl or a boy (Seavey et al., 1975; Sidorowicz & Lunney, 1980). Boy babies are described as "big" and "strong" and are bounced and handled more physically than girl babies who are described as "pretty" and "sweet" and are handled more gently. Even before birth, after finding out their child's sex via ultrasound, parents describe their girls-to-be as "finer" and "quieter" than boys-to-be, who are described as "more coordinated." By 1 month of age, mothers tend to rate their sons, and fathers tend to rate their daughters, less positively. Moreover, mothers and fathers alike tend to view their 4-month-old daughters in more negative terms when they cried, but no such negative perceptions emerged when sons cried. In fact, more crying by boys was associated with mothers' tendency to rate their sons as more powerful, whereas more crying by daughters was associated with mothers' tendencies to rate their daughters as less powerful. Similar biases are evident in other appraisals of infants. Mothers of 11-month-old boys *over*estimated how well their babies would crawl down a sloped pathway, whereas mothers of 11-month-old girls *under*estimated how well their babies would do. Subsequent objective tests of crawling ability on the sloped path revealed no gender differences in infant crawling (Mondschein et al., 2000). Parents further tilt gender development in their children by tending to place girls and boys in gender-distinctive contexts, such as rooms with certain furnishings including dolls for girls and cars for boys. Nor are parents' opinions shaped by the behaviors of their girl or boy babies. Parents purchase gender-stereotyped toys for their children a few months before the child's birth, well prior to when children could express gender-typed toy preferences themselves.

In these and other ways, parents' sex-differentiated behaviors are robust and consistent. Parents are more likely to give boys traditional names and are more likely to name boys after a parent or relative. Girls are more likely to be given made-up names, and when a traditional boy name becomes commonly used for girls, the name no longer is given to boys (Evelyn used to be a boy's name). In addition, from birth onward, fathers appear to interact preferentially with sons and mothers with daughters, and the ways that mothers and fathers interact with their daughters and sons differ. Mothers are more likely to play with their girls with dolls and engage them in social pretense, whereas boys are encouraged to play with vehicles. Because social pretense elicits more complex language, questions, and descriptions about objects, from an early age parents likely provide their male and female infants with different cognitive experiences in addition to teaching them what types of toys are appropriate for boys and girls. Childcare providers also reinforce gender stereotypes by the types of activities they encourage, the toys they provide, and the comments they make, such as praising a girl for her appearance and a boy for his activity level.

Despite the vast similarities between the genders, gender stereotyping appears to take root quickly and robustly. Before infants are able to label themselves as a girl or a boy (an ability that emerges around age 2), girls have begun to prefer dolls and boys to prefer cars. Not unexpectedly, the effects of gender expectancies spill over to other spheres of development. Infants who acquire gender labels before the end of the second year (called "early labelers") are also more gender-typed in their toy choices than are late labelers. Moreover, parents' responses to infants' gender-typed play at 1½ years predict whether infants will be early or late in acquiring the ability to label gender. Parents of infants who label early give more attention (both positive and negative) when their children play with either male- or female-gender-typed toys, regardless of the child's actual gender.

INFANT–SIBLING AND INFANT–PEER RELATIONSHIPS

INFANTS' RELATIONSHIPS WITH SIBLINGS

According to the U.S. Census Bureau, approximately 80% of parents in the United States have more than one child. This means that most infants have an older sibling or have or are going to have a younger sister or brother. Relationships between infants and their siblings are complex and factors of age, spacing, gender, and culture all play parts in their nature. On the one hand, infant–sibling relationships are more alike, have more interests in common, and are more similar in their behavioral capacities than infant–adult relationships. On the other hand, siblings resemble infant–adult pairs in that siblings differ in cognitive and social abilities and experiences. Also, two sisters and two brothers may have much in common, whereas opposite-sex siblings very little. Siblings close in age and therefore spacing, may be more alike than siblings who differ a lot in age. In Western industrialized societies, older siblings are infrequently entrusted

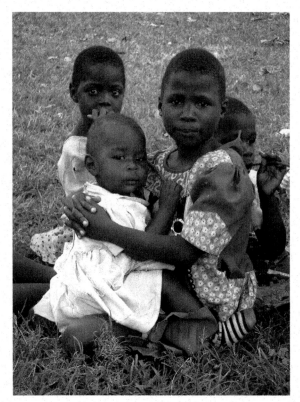

Figure 6.3 In some cultures, older siblings look after their younger siblings, thus allowing their parents to work and manage the household. (Image Courtesy of Shutterstock, Inc. Copyright: Steffen Foerster/Shutterstock.com.)

with actual caring for a younger infant in the family. In many non Western countries, by contrast, older siblings often assume major responsibilities for infant care (Figure 6.3).

These similarities and differences help to define how younger and older siblings relate to one another. For example, older siblings tend to be more dominant, assertive, and directing than younger siblings. They may spend time teaching skills to their younger siblings. Reciprocally, infant siblings are well known to monitor what their older siblings are doing, attempting to imitate or explore the toys just abandoned by an older sister or brother. This imitation strategy optimizes what infants learn about the environment. Children with siblings understand others' perspectives in the theory-of-mind sense better and earlier. In these ways, although older siblings are not charged with formal childcare responsibilities, older siblings still influence the cognitive and social skills of infants through informal combinations of teaching and modeling.

Just as parental (marital) relationships affect parent–child relationships, parent–child and parent–parent relationships also influence sibling relationships. Infants who have secure attachments with their mothers protest less and are less aggressive when their mothers play with their older siblings. For their part, preschoolers who are securely attached to their mothers are more likely to respond to the distress of their infant siblings by being nurturing. Siblings are also more positive toward each other when both enjoy nurturant relationships with their fathers. In addition, the quality of the parental marriage affects sibling relationship quality (among other things, see Box 6.3). European American, Mexican American, and Taiwanese mothers who report higher levels of marital satisfaction also report positive sibling relationships in their children (Yu & Gamble, 2008). Positivity begets positivity, and not unexpectedly high-quality sibling relationships promote positive parenting. In the broader family constellation, sibling relationships are more

BOX 6.3   Exposure to Domestic Violence Alters Infants' Reaction to Conflict

Does experience with interpersonal or domestic violence influence the way infants respond to conflict? In one study, 12-month-olds were exposed to an adult having a scripted 30-second telephone argument (Dejonghe et al., 2005). After the argument, the adult played with the infant for 5 minutes, during which time infants were rated for their degree of distress relying on facial, vocal, and postural expressions. Mothers also completed a temperament questionnaire. Thirty of the 89 infants had mothers who reported experiencing domestic violence within the infants' lifetime. Infants exposed to domestic violence showed significantly higher levels of distress compared to infants who did not have experience with domestic violence. However, infants without a history of domestic violence showed different levels of distress depending on their temperament. Infants who were judged to be temperamentally more active, less adaptable, and more likely to express negative mood showed greater distress than calmer, more adaptable, and easy infants. Thus, exposure to domestic violence seems to elevate a child's later distress response to conflict, and this effect is above and beyond different temperament. Does this mean that children who witness interpersonal violence are affected long term? The answer is yes. Muller and Tronick (2019) proposed that effects of exposure to domestic violence are long lasting. Witnessing domestic violence can permanently alter both structure and function in infancy.

prosocial when parent–child relationships and parents' marriages are reported as high quality, and especially when parents do not treat siblings differently. It is understandably difficult for parents with two young children to be strictly even handed. Having one child, a parent can devote as much or as little time, attention, and effort as the parent wishes. Having two children necessarily divides a parent's time, attention, and effort. Parents with a second child are already older than they were with their first, which may tax the parent-infant relationship, yet they also have more experience, which may benefit the parent–infant relationship. On the one hand, parents know more about parenting by the time a second infant comes along; on the other hand, parents of a second born show lower levels of engagement, such as physical encouragement, social exchange, and language, than they did with their first born – even when they are alone with the second born (Bornstein et al., 2019).

INFANTS' RELATIONSHIPS WITH PEERS

Infants who do not have older siblings are only exposed to other children when they enroll in an alternative care setting or an informal play group. As dual wage earner families have become the norm in many societies, increasing numbers of infants spend extended periods of time in relationships with unrelated children. Infants' exposure to a variety of other children who have different behavioral styles and provide contrasting patterns of interaction fosters the development of a more sophisticated and flexible repertoire of social skills. Indeed, interaction with other children during infancy has long been judged to constitute a vital ingredient of social development. For example, peer interactions afford infant rhesus monkeys opportunities to learn how to play, how to fight, how to relate to members of the opposite sex, and how to communicate with other monkeys (Figure 6.4). When deprived of peer interaction, infant monkeys grow into socially incompetent adults.

Infant–peer relationships develop in stages. Very young infants show an interest in peers, but social interactions between infants in the first half year of life are infrequent, and when they occur they are usually brief. By 6 months, infants may initiate exchanges and respond to one another's social overtures with combinations of looks, smiles, and vocalizations. From 6 to 12 months, infant–peer interactions may increase, and responsiveness to peer overtures and imitation become more common. Between 12 and 18 months, infants become aware of their feelings and realize that others have feelings as well, so empathic and prosocial behaviors make their

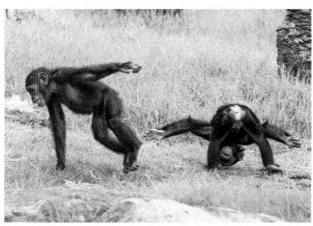

Figure 6.4 Primate peers playing. Such interactions are important in the social development of young primates and human infants. (Image Courtesy of Shutterstock, Inc. Copyright: Andy333/Shutterstock.com.)

appearance. By 2 years of age, helping, giving, and sharing are common, and infants have been observed attempting to respond to a peer's negative emotions by offering a toy or alerting an adult that another child is upset.

Some infants simply prefer to play by themselves, but others are sociable. One study recorded peer interactions in infants between 12 and 17 months of age in a childcare setting (Williams et al., 2007). Three kinds of social competence were observed. Peer sociability included smiling at peers, initiating play, and taking toys from peers. Active peer refusal included refusing peers' attempts to play, turning one's back on peers, and physically moving away from peers. Passive peer avoidance included watching rather than participating and acting as though not noticing peers' attempts to initiate play. Among infants (as opposed to older children), taking a toy away from another child is not necessarily a hostile act, but may obliquely indicate a desire for social interaction. Other acts, like hitting or biting can be ways infants actively avoid interactions.

Developmental scientists agree that children who have secure relationships with their parents should be sociable and socially competent with peers. Infants with warm, sensitive parents who grow up in harmonious families are indeed better adjusted socially, unaggressive, and popular. However, parent–child relationships are not the only family factors that affect infants' peer relationships. In addition to positive socialization practices they have experienced within the family, infants' interactions with peers likewise reflect their own social, cognitive, and emotional attainments As infants likely come into contact with peers in formal and informal contexts of childcare, helpful and sensitive caregivers also monitor and respond to their individual differences, encouraging infants to join a peer group, directing and talking about other children, objects, clothing, feelings, and intentions, and moderating infants' potentially negative peer relationships by distracting infants from other children or objects (Williams et al., 2010).

NONPARENTAL CARE

A greater understanding of infancy acknowledges the richness, diversity, and complexity of infants' early experiences involving all family members. Well over one-half of infants in the United States spend most of their week in nonparental care, and so these relationships too merit attention. Families of all kinds want or need to use supplementary care for their infants, often driven by economic concerns and motives such as mothers in the workforce or pursuing a career. In addition, many infants across the world live in multigeneration families, where the burden of infant care may be shared among parents, grandparents, aunts, uncles, and cousins.

In practice, nonparental care arrangements take a bewildering array of forms, and any individual infant may follow an equally bewildering course of care on their way to their second birthday. In the United States, perhaps 30% of children are in center-based care (called "daycare"), 25% in non relative home-based care, and 45% with another relative, such as a grandparent or sibling. The number of hours infants spend in nonmaternal care varies considerably by child age: fewer hours as newborns, more hours as toddlers. Furthermore, the nature and quality of nonparental care vary widely across centers, homes, and babysitters. This variability, combined with the fact that the values, practices, and economic profiles of parents who do or do not enroll their infants in nonparental care differ, render reckoning the effects of infant care on developing children almost impossible and generalizations risky.

One advantage conferred by nonparental care is that it allows infants to experience relationships with adults other than parents. These relationships can share some important features with infants' relationships with parents, especially when care providers are warm, sensitive, and nurturant as parents might be. However, nonparental care providers, especially in childcare centers, are charged with responsibilities for many children at once and so the individualized care an infant might enjoy with mother alone is out of the question. Rather, group interactions dominate in childcare centers. Even when care providers are engaged in one-on-one interaction with individual infants, they oversee the rest of the group too. In consequence, infants need to learn to wait and delay gratification.

How infants adjust to nonparental care may be related to their attachment security to their parents, with infants who enjoy secure attachments faring better than those with insecure attachments. Likewise, mothers who are more emotionally available to their infants have children who are better equipped to deal with stressful circumstances, like the transition to daycare. To help infants adjust, many European daycare centers implement adaptation programs in which mothers accompany infants during a transitional period of enrollment.

It is common for parents to choose group care arrangements, such as daycare, in the belief that peer interactions play a facilitative role in infants' social development, especially fostering the development of empathy and the acquisition of social skills. However, large-scale studies suggest that more nonmaternal care in the first 4½ years of life predicts more behavior problems (assertiveness, disobedience, and aggression) displayed at home or in the first year of formal schooling and that these problems persist up into adolescence (Burchinal et al., 2015; McCartney et al., 2010). Full-day placement in daycare may be physiologically and emotionally stressful for many, if not most, infants, and some negative effects of daycare are thought to be attributable to infants and children having trouble adjusting to that stress (Drugli et al., 2018). The general story for cognitive development in infants in daycare is more optimistic, especially among infants from low-income resource-deprived families who attend stimulating and enriching daycare programs. Children from well-resourced backgrounds do not consistently profit from daycare as much, presumably because they enjoy stimulating and enriching environments at home, but many children attending daycare from resourced-deprived circumstances show cognitive advantages over children cared for at home. At the end of the day, family factors, such as parental education and secure attachments, are more robust predictors of children's longer-term development than the quality or type of nonparental care a child has experienced growing up.

SOCIAL CLASS, ETHNICITY, CULTURE, AND TIME

At the start of this chapter, we introduced Bioecological Systems Theory. The chapter first focused on microsystems that infants experience directly and infants' immediate social partners – parents, siblings, peers, and nonparental caregivers. What about more macrosystems – social class, ethnicity, culture – and the chronosystem of time? Everyone belongs to a social class, ethnicity, and culture, and everyone lives at a certain point in time. How do these distal systems affect infant development?

SOCIAL CLASS

Social class (*aka* socioeconomic status) is indexed by three quantitative factors: parents' education, occupation, and income. Normally, parents try to instill values that will maximize their children's chances of success in the social class in which their children are likely to find themselves as mature adults. Professional-class parents in Western industrialized societies expect that their children will hold positions of responsibility; they therefore emphasize self-reliance, independence, autonomy, creativity, and curiosity, and expect their children to master academic-related skills (Farkas, 2018). By contrast, working-class parents expect their children to have as little opportunity for self-actualization and leadership as they themselves had, and they tend to emphasize obedience and conformity, values that will maximize their children's chances of success in the roles they are expected to fill in society. These generalized predictions are borne out in differences in the very language professional-class versus working-class mothers use with their infants. Even though infants are not yet talking themselves, professional-class mothers tend to talk to their babies more and acknowledge their infants' actions promoting effectance, whereas working-class mothers talk less and limit their utterances to directions and corrections.

Poverty and extreme economic disadvantage affect infant development in ways that go well beyond maternal speech patterns, values, and expectations. Just under one-half of children in the United States live in low-income families and almost one-quarter live in families whose income falls below the federal poverty level (currently $23,030 for a family of 3). Growing up lacking resources even for basic needs, such as food, clothing, clean water, and proper shelter, profoundly affects children's development. Generally speaking, infants living in poverty experience lower levels of emotional and verbal responsiveness, enjoy fewer opportunities for variety in daily stimulation and possess fewer appropriate play materials, and live in more chaotic, disorganized, and unstructured environments than infants from better-resourced homes (Magnuson & Duncan, 2019).

ETHNICITY

Ethnicity defines a grouping of people who identify with each other on the basis of shared attributes, such as a common set of traditions, ancestry, language, history, society, culture, nation, religion, or social treatment within their residing area, and distinguishes their group from other groups. In the United States, the U.S. Census broadly distinguishes European American, Latin American, African American, and Asian American ethnicities as well as other less populous ones like Pacific Islanders. People of different ethnicities often think about and treat infants of their ethnicity differently from those of other ethnicities. For example, African American, Mexican immigrant, Dominican immigrant, and Chinese immigrant mothers in the United States hold very different expectations for their newborn babies (Tamis-LeMonda & Kahana-Kalman, 2009). Within hours of giving birth, mothers in these groups were asked three questions: (1) How do you think things will change in your life and your family now that you have a baby? (2) What are your hopes and plans for your child and family over the next year? (3) Do you have any concerns right now about your child or family? Mothers' responses to these open-ended questions were coded with respect to four general categories: child development, parenting, family, and resources. New mothers' concerns focused most on resources and least on child development. However, African American and Dominican immigrant mothers were the most concerned with the issue of resources, and many of their answers pertained to rearing their children in a better environment. Chinese immigrant mothers focused the most on child development, especially in the context of their child's future education. Mexican immigrant mothers spoke most about family.

A study of Mexican and Dominican families in New York City teaches several lessons about ethnic variation in parenting practices. The two Latin American groups were similarly Spanish-speaking, hailed largely from low-socioeconomic status homes in the same city, and were parenting infants of the same age, but they and their infants still differed in meaningful ways in immigration patterns, levels of social isolation, residential stability, and poverty rate. Mexican infants had larger receptive vocabularies at 14 months of age, and Dominican infants had larger productive vocabularies at 24 months of age. Although Mexican and Dominican mothers reported growing up speaking Spanish, Dominican mothers spoke more English during literacy activities with their infants than did Mexican mothers, who spoke more Spanish. Thus, not all members of even similar immigrant groups share the same ideas or practices regarding parenting infants. Additionally, Dominican immigrant mothers and Mexican immigrant mothers engaged in different amounts of emotional support with their children. Similarly, when Québécois, Haitian, and Vietnamese mothers, all living in Montréal, were asked about the physical and social environment they provided for their infant, their perceptions and beliefs concerning infant development, and their interaction patterns with their infants, Pomerleau and colleagues (1991) unearthed cultural differences in the organization of the physical and social milieux parents provided, in maternal beliefs, as well as in behavioral strategies in interactions and teaching. When mothers were asked to report the age at which they consider that infants acquire various perceptual, cognitive, social, and motor abilities, for example, 16 of 19 domains showed differences among the groups.

In the United States, there are professional-class African Americans and European Americans just as there are working-class African Americans and European Americans. Ethnicity and social class both are influential in infant development and parent–infant interactions. In one study, low- and middle-class African American and European American families with 3- to 4-month-old infants were observed for 12 hours a day for 4 days (Fouts et al., 2012). Socioeconomic status differences in maternal and paternal holding, maternal carrying, and paternal caregiving emerged (Figure 6.5), and ethnic differences in maternal availability, affection, caregiving, and stimulation emerged. Such findings indicate that socioeconomic status and ethnicity have independent effects on infancy and infant development.

CULTURE

An anthropologist once profoundly observed to one of us [Bornstein] that the most important thing in a child's life is the country where the child is born. There is a great deal of truth in this statement. Consider two infants: One is born into a traditional group of nomadic hunter-gatherers, living in temporary homes, and spending much of each day in large communal multi-age groups occupied with obtaining food. The other is born into a modern Western culture, isolated most of the day at home with a single adult caregiver, whose food is purchased, and who comes into contact with few other people who show little interest in the infant's welfare. Cultural differences in worldview influence the frequency with which infants are cared for by mothers, other children, or unrelated adults, the extent to which infants are allowed to explore, and whether infants' experiences are nurturing or restrictive.

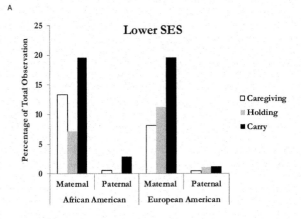

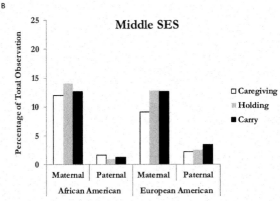

Figure 6.5 Percentages of time lower-SES (A) and middle-SES (B) African American and European American mothers and fathers engaged in caregiving activities, holding, and carrying their 3- to 4-month-old infants. Differences between mothers and fathers vary as a function of both SES and ethnicity. (Created by M. E. Arterberry from data in Fouts et al., 2012.)

For example, infant–mother sleeping arrangements result from very different cultural norms and customs. In some cultures, infants sleep in separate rooms from parents, whereas others practice parent-infant co-sleeping. It is hardly necessary to rehearse that different cultures exert pervasive and lifelong influences on human development.

Cross-cultural developmental science has proven valuable to understanding infancy and infant development for many reasons. First, people are always curious about development in cultures not their own, and anthropologists have regularly reported about vast differences in childhood and childcare in the (usually exotic) cultures they study. Second, understanding development in our own culture improves as a consequence of becoming aware of alternative developmental trajectories in other cultures. Third, more completely understanding development itself depends on seeing how development unfolds across a wide spectrum of contexts. (Like the proverbial fish in water, it is sometimes not possible to see what factors affect development when immersed in those factors, but they become clear when they are absent in other cultures.) Fourth, knowing what is ordinary and normative and what is extraordinary and non normative comes from exposure to the full range of human experience. Last, cross-cultural research permits tests of the commonalities versus specificities of structures and functions.

Viewing infant development from the perspective of only a single culture can lead to significant errors in understanding infancy and human development. An informative example comes from motor development in infancy. Recall from Chapter 2 that the pediatrician Gesell documented physical (and psychological) development in infancy and constructed detailed "cinematic atlases" of "normal development" on the basis of which he confidently offered "developmental diagnoses" of the progress and prognosis of normal and abnormal infant development. But Gesell based his research exclusively on infants and families in the United States, and only later did infant testing reach beyond middle-class European American families that Gesell studied. The results of cross-cultural comparisons with Native Americans and peoples in Africa and Southeast Asia showed that babies deviate from the accepted norms for European Americans with respect to the stages and the timing of motor development. When Bornstein and his colleagues (2017) videorecorded interactions of almost 800 mothers and their 5-month babies in 11 different countries (Argentina, Belgium, Brazil, Cameroon, France, Israel, Italy, Japan, Kenya, South Korea, and the United States), detailed coding revealed cultural variation in most infant and maternal behaviors. Infants differed in the extent to which they engaged in physical, social, and exploration activities as well as how much they vocalized nondistress, and mothers engaged in different amounts of physical, social, and teaching behaviors. Moreover, mothers provided different material resources to their infants, and they spoke to their infants in different amounts. Notably, certain infant and mother behaviors related to each other: Mothers who promoted physical development in their babies had babies who achieved higher levels of physical development, mothers who engaged their babies more in mutual interactions had infants who engaged with them socially more, and mothers who encouraged their infants' attention to objects, properties, and events in the environment more and out-fitted their infants' surroundings more had babies who attended to the environment more. Such cultural differences in so basic a realm of infant development reminds us that we need to more and more appreciate, rather than denigrate, cultural differences.

Earlier in this chapter, we described infant-parent attachment classifications in U.S. samples. One of Bowlby's hypotheses regarding attachment is its universality, referring to the fact that all infants come into the world with the wherewithal to form attachments. Does attachment develop the same way in different cultures despite wide variation in caregiving? Are the distributions of attachment classifications the same across cultures? Figure 6.6 displays the distributions of infants across three attachment categories in several countries. Most infants in all countries are securely attached, but there is considerable variation across countries in the percentages of infants classified as insecure-avoidant and insecure-resistant. These results could mean that parents in the six cultures are either more or less sensitive, or the results could reveal that factors other than the quality of parenting explain attachment (including behavior in the Strange Situation). For example, Japanese and Israeli babies are

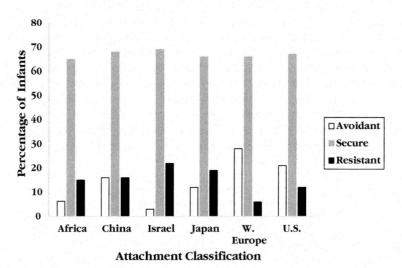

Figure 6.6 Percentages of infants classified as insecure-avoidant, secure, and insecure-resistant from 39 samples across six countries. (Created by M. E. Arterberry using data from van IJzendoorn & Sagi-Schwartz, 2008.)

notably stressed by the Strange Situation which may be responsible for higher proportions of Japanese and Israeli infants being classified as insecure-resistant. Japanese infants might be distressed because they typically have much less experience being separated from their mothers than infants from other cultures, or because their mothers are more stressed by the Strange Situation procedure and their infants are simply responding to their mothers' stress. Thus, the Strange Situation procedure may be structurally the same for infants from different cultures, but the psychological experience or meaning for infants from each culture may be very different.

The story of cross-cultural developmental science is one of differences but also similarities. Examples of commonalities across cultures are equally illuminating to understanding infancy. Not all infant and maternal behaviors Bornstein and his colleagues (2017) coded in the 11 cultures above differed. One baby and one mother behavior were each remarkably similar across cultures. Among infants, amounts of distress vocalizations (cries) were the same; infants' cries as cues to caregiving are vital to infants' survival and thriving. Among mothers, the amounts of nurturance (feeding, grooming, clothing) were the same; to survive and thrive, all babies must be nurtured in these ways. A second example is conversation. As noted in Chapter 4, in a conversational exchange between two people, one person is quiet while the other person speaks, and the first person waits to speak until the other person stops speaking. That is, they take turns. Language and information exchange are so important that we might predict that conversational turn-taking must be acquired very early regardless of culture or language, and it is. From the 11-country study just referred to, Bornstein and his colleagues (2017) coded the vocal interactions of those 800 mothers and their 5-month-old babies. By analyzing the onsets and offsets of all mother and infant vocalizations, the researchers found turn-taking everywhere: The vast majority of mothers began to speak to their infants within 2 seconds of their infants ceasing to vocalize and that more than half of the 5-month-olds likewise began to vocalize within 2 seconds of their mothers stopping to speak to them.

Cross-cultural developmental science has largely focused on comparing infancy and parenting in families living in two or more countries. Since 2000, many millions of families world-wide have left their home country and moved to a new one. Families migrate for many reasons – including economics, education, climate, famine, family reunification, and war – many, if not all, with the goal to provide a better life for their children (as the mass migration of Ukrainian mothers with young children in 2022 vividly demonstrated).

Families face many challenges in adjusting to a new culture, not the least of which is **acculturating** to new and different cultural customs and beliefs regarding the best way to rear infants.

Comparing immigrant families to each other and to families in their countries of origin and destination reveals that parenting cognitions and parenting practices are both affected by acculturation. For example, studies of Japanese American and South American families who had moved to the United States find that South American mothers engage in more social behavior, talk to their infants more, and provide more auditory stimulation in their infants' environment than do Japanese American mothers (Bornstein & Cote, 2001). Like their mothers, South American infants engage in more social behaviors than do Japanese American infants. Between cognitions and practices, parenting practices appear to acculturate more quickly or readily than parenting cognitions. In a number of domains (including personality, play, and other types of everyday behavior such as feeding), immigrant mothers show patterns that are more like those shown by mothers in the country of destination than like those shown in their country of origin.

Nations across the world are heterogeneous in that social class, ethnic, and cultural differences within and between nations generate and give meaning to childrearing. Social classes, ethnicities, and cultures vary with respect to the patterns of development they expect, encourage, and support. Class, ethnic, and cultural prescriptions determine, to a great extent, the immediate contexts infants experience, the short- and long-term goals parents have for their children, and the practices used by parents in efforts to meet those goals. The childrearing cognitions and practices of one's own class, ethnicity, or culture might seem normal, but some practices are actually rather unusual in a relative sense. For example, some cultures ensure that infants are reared in intimate extended families and cared for by many relatives; others isolate mothers and babies. Some assign complex and intimate responsibilities to fathers; others treat fathers as irrelevant social objects. In short, macrosystems play major roles in shaping infant development.

Class, ethnic, and cultural comparisons are valuable and informative, but "differences" are always tricky and need to be considered with a great deal of caution for a variety of reasons. One, there is always variability inside classes, ethnicities, and cultures. Infants always vary among themselves in growing, thinking, communicating, and feeling; likely, then, the distributions in different groups overlap quite a bit raising the question of whether any between-group difference is as important as within-group variability. Two, group differences are susceptible to unjust conclusions: group 1 (us) is different from group 2 (them), so group 1 is better than group 2. Three, samples in different groups can differ in a host of ways other than class, ethnicity, or culture: If mothers of two classes, ethnicities, and cultures differ in their parenting infants, are we sure that it was class, ethnicity, or culture that made the difference, and not a difference in, say, mothers' education?

HISTORICAL TIME

The anthropologist's observation that the most important thing in a child's life is *where* the child is born might be amended to include *when* the child was born. The sheer probability of surviving infancy has changed dramatically through history. In the year 1990, almost 9 million infants world-wide died in the first year of life; in 2017, that staggering number was reduced to 4 million. Before 1990, infant death was much more common: In the year 1800, almost one-half of children born did not live to see their fifth birthday.

Historical time permeates all sorts of issues surrounding infant care. Many parents of infants today wonder whether exclusive parental care of infants is best and what the effects of nonparental care of infants may be. History has something to say about these issues. In the era in which modern humans evolved, group care of infants was common ("it takes a village to raise a baby"), and aristocratic and affluent Europeans and North Americans since ancient times regularly depended on wet nurses, nannies, and governesses to care for infants. A biography of Darwin recounts that in the early 1800s Charles and his siblings were reared by a nanny, slept in a separate house from their parents, and were allowed finally to dine with adults in the family only when their feet could touch the floor while sitting at the dining room table.

Ideological beliefs current at a given time powerfully shape the social ecology of infancy. Most developmental scientists come from, or were trained in, middle-class Western backgrounds. It is hardly surprising that they have focused their attention on the childrearing practices of people like themselves. Unfortunately, this focus can lead to a violation of one of the cautions outlined above, namely the tendency to view the beliefs, practices, and experiences of those from other backgrounds as deficient, rather than just different. The short-sightedness of an ethnocentric perspective is illustrated by an historical analysis of social class differences in infant rearing. When the same values were held at different times by middle- and lower-class parents – say, a preference for bottle feeding versus breastfeeding – they were positively evaluated when held by middle-class parents and negatively evaluated when adopted by lower-class parents.

SUMMARY

Infants are prepared from birth to become social partners on account of their early developing neural, motor, and mental capabilities. Moreover, infants engage in behaviors, such as imitation, that facilitate their interactions with significant others. During their first months of life, infants transit stages in attachment development and generally form attachments during the second half of their first year with those adults with whom they have had most consistent, reliable, extended affirmative interactions. Individual differences in the security of attachment relationships appear to depend on the quality of infants' early interactions as well as infants' own temperament. Attachment is one of many examples of how parents exert direct and indirect effects on infant development. Other influences come from infants' wider social ecology – siblings, peers, daycare providers – as well as macrosystems in which infant development is embedded – social class, ethnicity, culture, and time.

7

CODA: APPRECIATING THE WHOLE CHILD

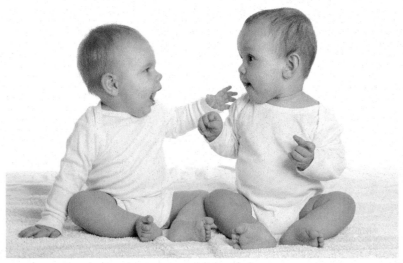

(Image courtesy of Shutterstock, copyright: Nina Anna/Shutterstock.com.)

INTRODUCTION

Infancy: The Basics is organized topically. Separate chapters are devoted to domains of growing, thinking, communicating, feeling, and relating. Each is a major substantive activity and accomplishment of infants, and so each merits separate discussion. However,

DOI: 10.4324/9781003172802-7

organizing the basics about infancy in this way obscures the genuine and intimate interrelatedness of these domains. This coda uses the development of social cognition in infancy to bring home the idea that growing, thinking, communicating, feeling, and relating in infants are integrated. That is, these different domains of development are related to one another in making a *whole child*. Illustrating this idea calls on material presented in earlier chapters. **Social cognition** refers to the ways that people perceive and understand their interactions with other people, come to know and rely on people with whom they interact, and appreciate differences between their own perspectives and knowledge and those of others.

DEVELOPMENT OF SOCIAL COGNITION

As infants come into the world and grow in independence, everything and everyone they naturally encounter is new and novel. To gain an understanding of what and who is safe and not, dependable, consistent, and responsive to their needs and not, infants call on their growing, thinking, communicating, feeling, and relating skills as well as the good-will and knowledge of their caregivers. Imagine an infant sitting in an infant seat or crawling on the floor, only to encounter an unfamiliar animated mechanical toy. The infant might be uncertain how to react. Growing allows the infant to react physically (approach or withdraw). Perceiving allows the infant to understand the toy's dimensions (size, color) and track the toy's movement (approach or away), and thinking allows the infant to decide about the toy's intentions and future action (harmless or potentially threatening). Communicating allows the infant to share reactions at a distance (giggle or cry). Feeling allows the infant to express emotions about the event (glee or fear). And relating allows the infant to involve others (to gain information and resolve any ambiguity associated with the novel toy). All these activities come together in **social referencing**, using others' emotional expressions to understand situations, including novel and ambiguous ones such as the mechanical toy in question. Social referencing itself encompasses awareness that adults may possess valuable knowledge that infants can access and use to help regulate their own emotions and reactions in such situations. A novel animated toy might present an intriguing sight; yet such toys might initially elicit wariness. If a parent appears fearful, the infant is likely to withdraw, but if the parent smiles and speaks in a friendly, supportive voice, the infant is likely to approach the toy to examine it more closely and engage with it.

Action, perception, cognition, emotion, communication, and relating are all at play. The infant must have the perceptual abilities to detect the toy and the affective expressions of the parent. To ensure that the parent's expression pertains to the toy in question, the infant must confirm that the parent is also oriented toward it. The infant must have the cognitive presence of mind to evaluate the situation, perhaps remembering similar situations in the past, and to seek clarifying information from the parent. The infant must have a sense of any emotions involved for themselves and in others as well as be able to communicate the significance of the event. The infant must have a sense of trust in a parent for otherwise the infant would not follow the parent's expressions. The infant must learn how to associate the toy with the emotional information the parent provided and so act toward toys and other novel objects now and in future encounters when parental guidance is not present.

Social referencing has powerful effects, not only on reactions to objects but also on social behavior, such as reactions to strangers. Infants in the middle of the first year often respond negatively to unfamiliar adults. This common reaction is understood as **stranger anxiety**. One interpretation, based on social referencing, is that strangers are somewhat uncertain and ambiguous stimuli for young infants, who turn to trusted adults for emotional information about them. Infants respond less negatively, and sometimes even positively, to strangers when parents first react positively to them. Thus, it is not the strangers' unfamiliarity per se that elicits fearfulness in infants, but the reactions of trusted adults who are socially referenced by uncertain infants. When adults are positive and sociable about strangers, infants are likely to respond with friendliness rather than fearfulness.

Through social cognition, infants have the opportunity to learn – to learn about themselves, about the material world, and about other people. Decisions about whom to trust build on earlier abilities of growing, thinking, communicating, feeling, and relating. (A helpful hint emerges from this simple observation about infants. Infants are constantly being introduced to new people – grandparents, aunts and uncles, cousins, parents' friends, and others. The good-willed impulse of these strangers is to immediately invade the infant's space. A subtle but safer strategy is to let the infant see and hear the person first interact warmly with a trusted parent.)

CONCLUSION

Infancy: The Basics introduces human development over approximately the first 2 years of life. The book is intended primarily to convey and instill an appreciation, and hopefully a sense of wonder, for what a remarkable period of life infancy really is. The newborn sleeps most of the day and cannot communicate well, if at all, but quickly grows into the curious toddler who appears never to stop talking or moving. The dynamic miracle of development is challenging for a parent to catch hold of: What once-captivated mother or father would not like to "freeze" their baby's development at some landmark moment – the first social smile, the first independent step, or the first word? Change in the child is equally challenging for the developmental scientist to capture empirically. So, a secondary purpose of *Infancy: The Basics* is to communicate an appreciation for the sophistication of the developmental science behind infancy, including infants' growing, thinking, communicating, feeling, and relating, and the creative methods developmental scientists have conjured and employed to pierce the mystery of infancy and unveil infants' many competencies.

Infancy: The Basics also illustrates several key themes that pervade the study and understanding of this formative period in human development: sensitive periods, the transaction of nature and nurture, stages of development, attachment, stability and continuity, information processing, the beginnings of language, and temperament to name but a few. Also considered are the wider contexts of infants' development – the roles of parents, siblings, childcare providers, and culture, for example. Moreover, several theoretical perspectives are brought to bear as lenses through which infancy is understood and appreciated. An especially significant theoretical and practical take-away falls out of the whole-child view, viz. that of developmental cascades (Oakes & Rakison, 2020). As the infant grows, thinks, communicates, feels, and relates, development and change in each domain reflects earlier developments and changes in the other domains and reverberates in future developments and changes in the other domains.

Infancy is the first phase of extrauterine life, and it makes sense that the start has implications for what comes next and perhaps for maturity. So, it is entirely understandable that growing, thinking, communicating, feeling, and relating in infancy foretell and have consequences for the psychology of later childhood, adolescence, and perhaps adulthood. As longitudinal research has flourished, such connections from infancy have become more firmly established. They also anticipate applied questions. For example, can optimal development be fostered in infancy and, if so, how? Expanding our knowledge of infancy and developmental processes is critical to answering such vital generational questions. It is trite to say, as scientists always do, that "more research is needed," but in this case the trite is true: Too little is still known about infants, and what infancy portends for later development, yet so much is at stake. Every house is constructed on a foundation and endures on the sturdiness of that foundation. Infants grow into voting, driving, reproducing citizens in, say, 18 short years. The more we know about brain development, the origins of thinking and language, the regulation of emotions, as well as how social and cultural contexts shape development from infancy, the better prepared we will be to help our voting, driving, reproducing children mature into the educated flourishing citizens we wish them to be. At the end of the day, understanding infancy and fostering optimal development from infancy turn on appreciating the whole child. In this grand sense, developmental science is indispensable and irreplaceable. Developmental science is the window on infant competencies – how they emerge and what makes them best – as well as how the complete and finished person first comes into being.

REFERENCES

Ainsworth, M. D. S., & Wittig, B. A. (1969). Attachment and exploratory behavior of one-year-olds in a strange situation. In B. M. Foss (Ed.), *Determinants of infant behavior* (Vol. 4, pp. 111–136). Routledge Methuen.

Anderson, D. R., & Pempek, T. A. (2005). Television and very young children. *American Behavioral Scientist, 48*(5), 505–522. http://dx.doi.org/10.1177/0002764204271506

Arterberry, M. E., & Bornstein, M. H. (2002). Infant perceptual and conceptual categorization: The roles of static and dynamic attributes. *Cognition, 86*, 1–24. http://dx.doi.org/10.1016/S0010-0277(02)00108-7

Arterberry, M. E., & Kellman, P. J. (2016). *Development of perception in infancy: The cradle of knowledge revisited*. Oxford University Press.

Baldwin, D. A., Markham, E. M., Bill, B., Desjardins, R. N., & Irwin, J. M. (1996). Infants' reliance on a social criterion for establishing word-object relations. *Child Development, 67*, 3135–3153. http://dx.doi.org/10.2307/1131771

Barr, R., Zack, E., Garcia, A., & Muentener, P. (2008). Infants' attention and responsiveness to television increases with prior exposure and parental interaction. *Infancy, 13*, 30–56. http://dx.doi.org/10.1080/15250000701779378

Baxter, J. (2011). Flexible work hours and other job factors in parental time with children. *Social Indicators Research, 101*, 239–242. http://dx.doi.org/10.1007/s11205-010-9641-4

Beier, J. S., & Spelke, E. S. (2012). Infants' developing understanding of social gaze. *Child Development, 83*(2), 486–496. http://dx.doi.org/10.1111/j.1467-8624.2011.01702.x

Bell, M. A. (2012). A psychobiological perspective on working memory performance at 8 months of age. *Child Development, 83*, 251–265. http://dx.doi.org/10.1111/j.1467-8624.2011.01684.x

Belsky, J., & Rovine, M. (1990). Q-sort security and first-year nonmaternal care. *New Directions for Child Development*, *49*, 7–22. http://dx.doi.org/10.1002/cd.23219904903

Benson, J. B., Cherry, S. S., Haith, M. M., & Fulker, D. W. (1993). Rapid assessment of infant predictors of adult IQ: Midtwin-midparent analyses. *Developmental Psychology*, *29*, 434–447. http://dx.doi.org/10.1037/0012-1649.29.3.434

Bernier, A., Ackerman, J. P., & Stovall-McClough, K. C. (2004). Predicting the quality of attachment relationships in foster care dyads from infants' initial behaviors upon placement. *Infant Behavior and Development*, *27*, 366–381. http://dx.doi.org/10.1016/j.infbeh.2004.01.001

Bertenthal, B. I., Proffitt, D. R., & Cutting, J. E. (1984). Infant sensitivity to figural coherence in biomechanical motions. *Journal of Experimental Child Psychology*, *37*, 213–230. http://dx.doi.org/10.1016/0022-0965(84)90001-8

Blasi, A., Mercure, E., Lloyd-Fox, S., Thomson, A., Brammer, M. Sauter, D., Deeley, Q., Barker, G. J., Renvall, V., Deoni, S., Gasston, D., Williams, S. C. R., Johnson, M H., Simmons A., & Murphy, D. G. M. (2011). Early specialization for voice and emotion processing in the infant brain. *Current Biology*, *21*, 1220–1224. http://dx.doi.org/10.1016/j.cub.2011.06.009

Booth, A. E., & Waxman, S. R. (2009). A horse of a different color: Specifying with precision infants' mappings of novel nouns and adjectives. *Child Development*, *80*, 15–22. http://dx.doi.org/10.1111/j.1467-8624.2008.01242.x

Bornstein, M. H. (2007). Hue categorization and color naming: Cognition to language to culture. In R. E. MacLaury, G. V. Paramei, & D. Dedrick (Eds.), *Anthropology of color: Interdisciplinary multilevel modeling* (pp. 3–27). John Benjamins.

Bornstein, M. H. (2009). Toward a model of culture-parent-child transactions. In A. Sameroff (Ed.), *The transactional model of development: How children and contexts shape each other* (pp. 139–161). American Psychological Association.

Bornstein, M. H. (2016). Determinants of parenting. In D. Cicchetti (Ed.), *Developmental psychopathology: Risk, resilience, and intervention* (pp. 180–270). John Wiley & Sons, Inc. http://dx.doi.org/10.1002/9781119125556.devpsy405

Bornstein, M. H. (2019). Parenting infants. In M. H. Bornstein (Ed.), *Handbook of parenting: Children and parenting* (Vol. 1, 3rd ed., pp. 3–55). Taylor & Francis Group.

Bornstein, M. H. (2022). *Parenting, infancy, and culture: Specificity in Argentina, Belgium, Israel, Italy, and the United States*. Routledge.

Bornstein, M. H., & Arterberry, M. E. (2003). Recognition, categorization, and apperception of the facial expression of smiling by 5-month-old infants. *Developmental Science*, *6*, 585–599. http://dx.doi.org/10.1111/1467-7687.00314

Bornstein, M. H., & Arterberry, M. E. (2010). The development of object categorization in young children: Hierarchical inclusiveness, age, perceptual attribute and group versus individual analyses. *Developmental Psychology*, *46*, 350–365. http://dx.doi.org/10.1037/a0018411

Bornstein, M. H., Arterberry, M. E., Mash, C., & Manian, N. (2011). Discrimination of facial expressions by 5-month-old infants of nondepressed and clinically depressed mothers. *Infant Behavior and Development*, *34*, 100–106. http://dx.doi.org/10.1016/j.infbe h.2010.10.002

Bornstein, M. H., & Cote, L. R. (2001). Mother-infant interaction and accultura-tion I: Behavioral comparisons in Japanese American and South American families. *International Journal of Behavioral Development, 25*, 549–563. http://dx. doi.org/10.1080/01650250042000546

Bornstein, M. H., Cote, L. R., Maital, S., Painter, K., Park, S., Pascual, L., Pecheux, M.-G., Ruel, J., Venuti, P., & Vyt, A. (2004). Cross-linguistic anal-ysis of vocabulary in toddlers: Spanish, Dutch, French, Hebrew, Italian, Korean, and English. *Child Development, 75*, 1115–1139. http://dx.doi. org/10.1111/j.1467-8624.2004.00729.x

Bornstein, M. H., Hahn, C.-S., & Wolke, D. (2013). Systems and cascades in cog-nitive development and academic achievement. *Child Development, 84*, 154–162. http://dx.doi.org/10.1111/j.1467-8624.2012.01849.x

Bornstein, M. H., & Mash, C. (2010). Experience-based and on-line categoriza-tion of objects in early infancy. *Child Development, 81*, 884–897. http://dx.doi. org/10.1111/j.1467-8624.2010.01440.x

Bornstein, M. H., Mash, C., Arterberry, M. E., & Manian, N. (2012). Object per-ception in 5-month-old infants of clinically depressed and nondepressed mothers. *Infant Behavior and Development, 35*, 150–157. http://dx.doi.org/ 10.1016/j.infbeh.2011.07.008

Bornstein, M. H., Putnick, D. L., Cote, L. R., Haynes, O. M., & Suwalsky, J. T. D. (2015). Mother-infant contingent vocalizations in 11 countries. *Psychological Science, 26*, 1272–1284. https://doi.org/10.1177/0956797615586796

Bornstein, M. H., Putnick, D. L., & Suwalsky, J. T. D. (2019). Mother-infant inter-actions with firstborns and secondborns: A within-family study of European Americans. *Infant Behavior and Development, 55*, 100–111. http://dx.doi.org/ 10.1016/j.infbeh.2019.03.009

Bornstein, M. H., Putnick, D. L., Yoonjung, P., Suwalsky, J. T. D., & Haynes, O. M. (2017). Human infancy and parenting in global perspective: Specificity. *Proceedings of the Royal Society B: Biological Sciences, 284*, 1–10. http://dx.doi. org/10.1098/rspb.2017.2168

Bowlby, J. (1969). *Attachment and loss: Attachment* (2nd ed., Vol. 1). Basic Books.

Boysson-Bardies, B., Sagart, L., & Durand, C. (1984). Discernible differences in the babbling of infants according to target language. *Journal of Child Language, 11*(1), 1–15. http://dx.doi.org/10.1017/S0305000900005559

Bridgett, D. J., Gartstein, M. A., Putnam, S. P., McKay, T., Iddins, E., Robertson, C., Ramsay, K., & Rittmueller, A. (2009). Maternal and con-textual influences and the effect of temperament development during infancy on parenting in toddlerhood. *Infant Behavior & Development, 32*, 103–116. http://dx.doi.org/10.1016/j.infbeh.2008.10.007

Bridgett, J. D., Ganiban, J. M., Neiderhiser, J. M., Natsuaki, M. N., Shaw, D. S., Reiss, D., & Leve, L. D. (2018). Contributions of mothers' and fathers' parenting to children's self-regulation: Evidence from an adoption study. *Developmental Science, 21*, 1–11. http://dx.doi.org/10.1111/desc.12692

Brooks, P., & Tomasello, M. (1998). How children avoid overgeneralization errors when acquiring transitive and intransitive verbs. In R. Brooks & M. Tomasello (Eds.), *The proceedings of the twenty-ninth annual child language research forum* (pp. 171–179). Center for the Study of Language and Information.

Burchinal, M., Magnuson, K., Powell, D., & Hong, S. S. (2015). Early childcare and education. In M. H. Bornstein, T. Leventhal, & R. Lerner (Eds.), *Handbook of child psychology and developmental science: Ecological settings and processes* (Vol. 4, 7th ed., pp. 223–267). Wiley.

Buss, A. H., & Plomin, R. (1984). *Temperament: Early developing personality traits.* Erlbaum.

Campos, J. J., Anderson, D. I., Barbu-Roth, M. A., Hubbard, W. M., Hertenstein, M. J., & Wirtherington, D. (2000). Travel broadens the mind. *Infancy, 1,* 149–219. http://dx.doi.org/10.1207/S15327078IN0102_1

Camerota, M. & Willoughby, M. T. (2021). Applying interdisciplinary frameworks to study prenatal influences on child development. *Child Development Perspectives, 15,* 24–30. https://doi.org/10.1111/cdep.12395

Camras, L. A., Perlman, S. B., Fries, A. B. W., & Pollak, S. D. (2006). Post-institutionalized Chinese and East European children: Heterogeneity in the development of emotion understanding. *International Journal of Behavioral Development, 30,* 193–199. http://dx.doi.org/10.1177%2F0165025406063608

Conboy, B. T., & Mills, D. L. (2006). Two languages, one developing brain: Event-related potentials to words in bilingual toddlers. *Developmental Science, 9,* F1–F12. http://dx.doi.org/10.1111/j.1467-7687.2005.00453.x

Cook, V., & Bassetti, B. (2011). *Language and bilingual cognition.* Psychology Press.

Darwin, C. R. (1859). *On the origin of species.* John Murray.

Darwin, C. R. (1872/1975). *The expression of the emotions in man and animals.* University of Chicago Press.

Darwin, C. R. (1877). A biographical sketch of an infant. *Mind, 2,* 286–294.

DeFries, J. C., Fulker, D. W., & LaBuda, M. C. (1987). Evidence for a genetic aetiology in reading disability of twins. *Nature, 329,* 537–539. http://dx.doi.org/10.1038/329537a0

De Houwer, A. *Bilingual Development in Childhood.* In M. H. Bornstein (Series Editor), *Cambridge Elements in Child Development.* Cambridge University Press, 2021. doi:10.1017/9781108866002

Dejonghe, E. S., Bogat, G. A., Levendosky, A. A., Von Eye, A., & Davidson, W. S. (2005). Infant exposure to domestic violence predicts heightened sensitivity to adult verbal conflict. *Infant Mental Health Journal, 26,* 268–281. http://dx.doi.org/10.1002/imhj.20048

Del Giudice, M., Ellis, B. J., & Shirtcliff, E. A. (2011). The adaptive calibration model of stress responsivity. *Neuroscience & Biobehavioral Reviews, 35,* 1562–1592. http://dx.doi.org/10.1016/j.neubiorev.2010.11.007

Deloache, J. S., Chiong, C. Sherman, K., Islam, N., Vanderborght, M., Troseth, G. L., Strouse, G. A., & O'Doherty, K. O. (2010). Do babies learn from baby media? *Psychological Science, 21,* 1570–1574. http://dx.doi.org/10.1177/0956797610384145

Dixon, W. E., & Smith, P. H. (2008). Attentional focus moderates habituation-language relationships: Slow habituation may be a good thing. *Infant and Child Development, 17,* 95–108. http://dx.doi.org/10.1002/icd.490

Dozier, M., Lindheim, O., Lewis, E., Bick, J., Bernard, K., & Peloso, E. (2009). Effects of a foster parent training program on young children's attachment behaviors: Preliminary evidence from a randomized clinical trial. *Child and Adolescence Social Work Journal, 26,* 321–332. https://doi.org/10.1007/s10560-009-0165-1

Drugli, M. B., Solheim, E., Lydersen, S., Vibeke, M., Smith, L., & Berg-Nielsen, T. S. (2018). Elevated cortisol levels in Norwegian toddlers in childcare. *Early Childhood Development and Care, 188,* 1684–1695. http://dx.doi.org/10.1080/03004430.2016.1278368

Else-Quest, N. M., Hyde, J. S., Goldsmith, H. H., & Van Hulle, C. A. (2006). Gender differences in temperament: A meta-analysis. *Psychological Bulletin, 132,* 33–72. http://dx.doi.org/10.1037/0033-2909.132.1.33

Fantz, R. L., Ordy, J. M., & Udelf, M. S. (1962). Maturation of pattern vision in infants during the first six months. *Journal of Comparative and Physiological Psychology, 55,* 907–917. https://psycnet.apa.org/doi/10.1037/h0044173

Farkas, G. (2018). Family, schooling, and cultural capital. In B. Schneider (Ed.), *Handbook of the sociology of education in the 21st century. Handbooks of sociology and social research* (pp. 3–38). Springer.

Farroni, T., Csibra, G., Simion, F., & Johnson, M. H. (2002). Eye contact detection in humans from birth. *Proceedings of the National Academy of Sciences, 99,* 9602–9605. http://dx.doi.org/10.1073/pnas.152159999

Fenson, L., Pethick, S., Renda, C., Cox, J. L., Dale, P. S., & Reznick, J. S. (2000). Short-form versions of the MacArthur communicative development inventories. *Applied Psycholinguistics, 21,* 95–116. http://dx.doi.org/https://doi.org/10.1017/S0142716400001053

Fernald, A. (2001). Hearing, listening, and understanding: Auditory development in infancy. In G. Bremner & A. Fogel (Eds.), *Blackwell handbook of infant development* (pp. 35–70). Blackwell.

Fraley, R. C. (2002). Attachment stability from infancy to adulthood: Meta-analysis and dynamic modeling of developmental mechanisms. *Personality and Social Psychology Review, 6,* 123–151.

Fransson, P., Skiöld, B., Horsch, S., Nordell, A., Blennow, M., Lagercrantz, H., & Åden, U. (2007). Resting-state networks in the infant brain. *Proceedings of the National Academy of Sciences, USA, 104,* 15531–15536. https://www.pnas.org/content/suppl/2007/09/25/0704380104.DC1

Frewen, P., Schroeter, M. L., Riva, G., Cipresso, P., Fairfield, B., Padulo, C., Kemp, A. H., Palaniyappan, L., Owolabi, M., Kusi-Mensah, K., Polyakova, M., Fehertoi, N., D'Andrea, W., Lowe, L., & Northoff, G. (2020). Neuroimaging the consciousness of self: Review, and conceptual-methodological framework. *Neuroscience & Biobehavioral Review, 112,* 164–212. http://dx.doi.org/10.1016/j.neubiorev.2020.01.023.

Friedrich, M., & Friederici, A. D. (2010). Maturing brain mechanisms and developing behavioral language skills. *Brain and Language, 114,* 66–71. http://dx.doi.org/10.1016/j.bandl.2009.07.004

Fouts, H. N., Roopnarine, J. L., Lamb, M. E., & Evans, M. (2012). Infant social interactions with multiple caregivers: The importance of ethnicity and socioeconomic status. *Journal of Cross-Cultural Psychology, 43,* 328–348. http://dx.doi.org/10.1177/0022022110388564

Gagne, J. R., & Goldsmith, H. H. (2011). A longitudinal analysis of anger and inhibitory control in twins from 12 to 36 months of age. *Developmental Science, 14*, 112–124. http://dx.doi.org/10.1111/j.1467-7687.2010.00969.x

Gartstein, M. A., Slobodskaya, H. R., Zylicz, P. O., Gosztyla, D., & Nakagawa, A. (2010). A cross-cultural evaluation of temperament: Japan, USA, Poland and Russia. *International Journal of Psychology and Psychological Therapy, 10*, 55–75.

Gattis, M. (2019). Parenting children born preterm. In M. H. Bornstein (Ed.), *Handbook of parenting. Vol. 1. Children and parenting* (3rd ed., pp. 424–466). Routledge.

Gibson, E. J., & Walk, R. D. (1960). The "visual cliff." *Scientific American, 202*, 64. http://dx.doi.org/10.1038/scientificamerican0460-64

Goldfield, B. A. (1985/86). Referential and expressive language: A study of two mother-child dyads. *First Language, 6*, 119–131. http://dx.doi.org/10.1177/014272378600601703

Goldin-Meadow, S. (2006). Nonverbal communication: The hand's role in talking and thinking. In W. Damon, D. Kuhn, & R. Siegler (Eds.), *The handbook of child psychology: Cognition, perception, and language* (6th ed., pp. 336–369). Wiley.

Goldstein, M. H., & Schwade, J. A. (2008). Social feedback to infants' babbling facilitates rapid phonological learning. *Psychological Science, 19*, 515–523. http://dx.doi.org/10.1111/j.1467-9280.2008.02117.x

Groh, A. M., Roisman, G. I., van IJzendoorn, M. H., Bakermans-Kranenburg, M. J., & Fearon, R. P. (2012). The significance of insecure and disorganized attachment for children's internalizing symptoms: A meta-analytic study. *Child Development, 83*, 591–610. http://dx.doi.org/10.1111/j.1467-8624.2011.01711.x

Hamlin, J. K. (2015). The case for social evaluation in preverbal infants: gazing toward one's goal drives infants' preferences for helpers over hinderers in the hill paradigm. *Frontiers in Psychology, 5*, 1563. 10.3389/fpsyg.2014.01563

Hamzelou, J. (2020). Coronavirus may cross placenta. *NewScientist, 246*(3282), 11. http://dx.doi.org/10.1016/S0262-4079(20)30911-8

Hebb, D. O. (1949). *The organization of behavior: A neuropsychology theory*. Wiley.

Hill-Soderlund, A. L., Mills-Koonce, W. R., Propper, C., Calkins, S. D., Granger, D. A., Moore, G. A., Gariepy, J.-L., & Cox, M. J. (2008). Parasympathetic and sympathetic responses to the strange situation in infants and mothers from avoidant and securely attached dyads. *Developmental Psychobiology, 50*, 361–376. http://dx.doi.org/10.1002/dev.20302

Hurtado, N., Marchman, V., & Fernald, A. (2008). Does input influence uptake? Links between maternal talk, processing speed and vocabulary size in Spanish-learning children. *Developmental Science, 11*, F31–F39. http://dx.doi.org/10.1111/j.1467-7687.2008.00768.x

Huttenlocher, P. R. (1990). Morphometric study of human cerebral cortex development. *Neuropsychologia, 28*, 517–527. http://dx.doi.org/10.1002/9780470753507.ch8

James, W. (1890). *The principles of psychology*. Henry Holt.

Johnson, M. H., Dziurawiec, S., Ellis, H., & Morton, J. (1991). Newborns' preferential tracking of face-like stimuli and its subsequent decline. *Cognition, 40,* 1–19. http://dx.doi.org/10.1002/9780470753507.ch8

Johnson, S. P., & Hannon, E. E. (2015). Perceptual development. In L. S. Liben, U. Müller, & R. M. Lerner (Eds.), *Handbook of child psychology and developmental science: Cognitive processes* (7th ed., vol. 2, pp. 63–112). Wiley.

Kagan, J., & Snidman, N. (2004). *The long shadow of temperament.* Harvard University Press.

Karasik, L. B., Adolph, K. E., Tamis-LeMonda, C. S., & Zuckerman, A. L. (2012). Carry on: Spontaneous object carrying in 13-month-old crawling and walking infants. *Developmental Psychology, 48,* 389–397. http://dx.doi.org/10.1037/a0026040

Keen, R. (2011). The development of problem solving in young children: A critical cognitive skill. *Annual Review of Psychology, 62,* 1–21.

Kerig, P. K. (2019). Parenting and family systems. In M. H. Bornstein (Ed.), *Handbook of parenting. Vol. 3. Being and becoming a parent* (3rd ed., pp. 3–35). Routledge.

Klein, R. G. (2011). Temperament: Half a century in the *Journal. Journal of the American Academy of Child & Adolescent Psychiatry, 50,* 1090–1092. http://dx.doi.org/10.1016/j.jaac.2010.07.013

Kovack-Lesh, K. A., McMurray, B., & Oakes, L. M. (2014). Four-month-old infants' visual investigation of cats and dogs: Relations with pet experience and attention strategy. *Developmental Psychology, 50,* 402–413. http://dx.doi.org/10.1037/a0033195

Kretch, K. S., & Adolph, K. E. (2013). Cliff or step? Posture-specific learning at the edge of a drop-off. *Child Development, 84,* 226–240. http://dx.doi.org/10.1111/j.1467-8624.2012.01842.x

Lee, J.-K., Schoppe-Sullivan, S. J., Feng, X., Gerhardt, M. L., & Kamp Dush, C. M. (2019). Advancing research and measurement on fathering and child development: III. Longitudinal measurement invariance across fathers' and mothers' reports of maternal gatekeeping behavior. *Monographs of the Society for Research in Child Development, 84,* 35–49. http://dx.doi.org/10.1002/mono.12404

Lewis, M. (2015). Emotional development and consciousness. In W. F. Overton, P. C. M. Molenaar, & R. M. Lerner (Eds.), *Handbook of child psychology and developmental science: Theory and method* (Vol. 1, 7th ed., pp. 407–451). Wiley.

Libertus, K., & Needham, A. (2010). Teach to reach: The effects of active vs. passive reaching experiences on action and perception. *Vision Research, 50,* 2750–2757. http://dx.doi.org/10.1016/j.visres.2010.09.001

Luke, B., & Brown, M. B. (2007). Elevated risks of pregnancy complications and adverse outcomes with increasing maternal age. *Human Reproduction, 22,* 1264–1272. http://dx.doi.org/10.1093/humrep/del522

Lyytinen, H., Ahonen, T., Eklund, K., Guttorm, T. K., Laakso, M.-L., Leinonen, S., Leppanen, P. H. T., Lyytinen, P., Poikkeus, A.-M., Puolakanaho, A., Richardson, U., & Viholainen, H. (2001). Developmental pathways of children with and without familial risk for dyslexia during the first years of life. *Developmental Neuropsychology, 20,* 535–554. http://dx.doi.org/10.1207/S15326942DN2002_5

Macken, M., & Barton, D. (1980). The acquisition of the voicing contrast in Spanish: A phonetic and phonological study of word-initial stop consonants. *Journal of Child Language, 7,* 433–458. http://dx.doi.org/10.1017/S0305000900002774

Magnuson, K. A., & Duncan, G. J. (2019). Parents in poverty. In M. H. Bornstein (Ed.), *Handbook of parenting. Vol. 4. Special conditions and applied parenting* (3rd ed., pp. 301–328). Routledge.

Main, M., & Cassidy, J. (1988). Categories of response to reunion with a parent at age six: Predicable from infant attachment classifications and stable over a one-month period. *Developmental Psychology, 24,* 415–426.

Mash, C., Arterberry, M. E., & Bornstein, M. H. (2007). Mechanisms of object recognition in 5-month-old infants. *Infancy, 12,* 31–43. http://dx.doi.org/10.1111/j.1532-7078.2007.tb00232.x

May, L. E., Glaros, A., Yeh, H. Clapp, J. F., & Gustafson, K. M. (2010). Aerobic exercise during pregnancy influences fetal cardiac autonomic control of heart rate and heart rate variability. *Early Human Development, 86,* 213–217. http://dx.doi.org/10.1016/j.earlhumdev.2010.03.002

McCartney, K., Burchinal, M., Clarke-Stewart, A., Bub, K. L., Owen, M. T., & Belsky, J. (2010). Testing a series of causal propositions relating time in child care to children's externalizing behavior. *Developmental Psychology, 46*(1), 1–17. http://dx.doi.org/10.1037/a0017886

McLaughlin, K. A., Sheridan, M. A., Tibu, F., Fox, N. A., Zeanah, C. H., & Nelson, C. A. (2015). Casual effects of the early caregiving environment on development of stress response systems in children. *Proceedings of the National Academy of Sciences, 112,* 5637–5642. http://dx.doi.org/10.1073/pnas.1423363112

Meltzoff, A. N., & Brooks, R. (2009). Social cognition and language. In J. Colombo, P. McCardle, & L. Freund (Eds.), *Infant pathways to language* (pp. 169–194). Psychology Press.

Meltzoff, A. N., & Moore, M. K. (1977). Imitation of facial and manual gestures by human neonates. *Science, 198,* 75–78. http://dx.doi.org/10.1126/science.198.4312.75

Meltzoff, A. N., Waismeyer, A., & Gopnik, A. (2012). Learning about causes from people: Observational causal learning in 24-month-old infants. *Developmental Psychology, 48*(5), 1215–1228. http://dx.doi.org/10.1037/a0027440.

Mondschein, E. R., Adolph, K. E., & Tamis-LeMonda, C. S. (2000). Gender bias in mothers' expectations about infant crawling. *Journal of Experimental Child Psychology, 77,* 304–316. http://dx.doi.org/10.1006/jecp.2000.2597

Moulson, M. C., Fox, N. A., Zeanah, C. H., & Nelson, C. A. (2009). Early adverse experiences and the neurobiology of facial emotional processing. *Developmental Psychology, 45,* 17–30. https://psycnet.apa.org/doi/10.1037/a0014035

Moulson, M. C., Westerlund, A., Fox, N. A., Zeanah, C. H., & Nelson, C. A. (2009). The effects of early experience on face recognition: An event-related potential study of institutionalized children in Romania. *Child Development, 80,* 1039–1056. http://dx.doi.org/10.1111/j.1467-8624.2009.01315.x

Muller, I., & Tronick, E. (2019). Early life exposure to violence: Developmental consequences on brain and behavior. *Frontiers in Behavioral Neuroscience, 13,* Article 156. http://dx.doi.org/10.3389/fnbeh.2019.00156

Murray, L., De Pascalis, L., Bozicevic, L., Hawkins, L., Sclafani, V., & Ferrari, P. F. (2016). The functional architecture of mother-infant communication, and the development of infant social expressiveness in the first two months. *Scientific Reports, 6.* http://dx.doi.org/10.1038/srep39019

Musso, D., Ko, A. I., & Baud, D. (2019). Zika virus infection—after the pandemic. *New England Journal of Medicine, 381*(15), 1444–1457. http://dx.doi.org/10.1056/NEJMra1808246

Myers, L. J., & Arterberry, M. E. (2022). Digital media and children under 3 years of age. *Infant Behavior and Development,* in press.

Nakanishi, R., & Imai-Matsumura, K. (2008). Facial skin temperature decreases in infants with joyful expression. *Infant Behavior and Development, 31,* 137–144. http://dx.doi.org/10.1016/j.infbeh.2007.09.001

Naoi, N., Minagawa-Kawai, Y., Kobayashi, A., Takeuchi, K., Nakamura, K., Yamamato, J., & Kojima, S. (2012). Cerebral responses to infant-directed speech and the effect of talker familiarity. *NeuroImage, 59,* 1735–1744. http://dx.doi.org/10.1016/j.neuroimage.2011.07.093

Nelson, C. A., Fox, N. A., & Zeanah, C. H. (2014). *Romania's abandoned children: Deprivation, brain development, and the struggle for recovery.* Harvard University Press.

Oakes, L. M., & Rakison, D. H. (2020). *Developmental cascades.* Oxford University Press.

Parke, R. D., & Cookston, J. T. (2019). Fathers and families. In M. H. Bornstein (Ed.), *Handbook of parenting: Being and becoming a parent* (Vol. 3, 3rd ed., pp. 64–136). Taylor & Francis Group.

Pasterski, V. L., Geffner, M. E., Brain, C., Hindmarsh, P., Brook, C., & Hines, M. (2005). Prenatal hormones and postnatal socialization by parents as determinants of male-typical toy plan in girls with congenital adrenal hyperplasia. *Child Development, 76,* 264–278. http://dx.doi.org/10.1111/j.1467-8624.2005.00843.x

Peltola, M. J., Strathearn, L., & Puurac, K. (2018). Oxytocin promotes face-sensitive neural responses to infant and adult faces in mothers. *Psychoneuroendocrinology* (91), 261–270. http://dx.doi.org/10.1016/j.psyneuen.2018.02.012

Piaget, J. (1952). *The origins of intelligence in children.* Norton.

Piaget, J. (1954). *The construction of reality in the child.* Basic Books. (Original work published 1937.)

Pivik, R. T., Andres, A., & Badger, T. M. (2011). Diet and gender influences on processing and discrimination of speech sounds in 3- and 6-month-old infants: A developmental ERP study. *Developmental Science, 14,* 700–712. http://dx.doi.org/10.1111/j.1467-7687.2010.01019.x

Pollak, S. D., Messner, M., Kistler, D. J., & Cohn, J. F. (2009). Development of perceptual expertise in emotion recognition. *Cognition, 110,* 242–247. http://dx.doi.org/10.1016/j.cognition.2008.10.010

Pomerleau, A., Malcuit, G., & Sabatier, C. (1991). Child-rearing practices and parental beliefs in these cultural groups of Montreal: Quebecois, Vietnamese,

Haitian. In M. H. Bornstein (Ed.), *Cultural Approaches to Parenting* (pp. 45–68). Lawrence Erlbaum.

Porter, R. H., Bologh, R. D., & Makin, J. W. (1988). Olfactory influences on mother-infant interactions. In C. Rovee-Collier & L. P. Lipsitt (Eds.), *Advances in infancy research* (Vol. 5, pp. 39–69). Ablex.

Pruden, S. M., Levine, S. C., & Huttenlocher, J. (2011). Children's spatial thinking: Does talk about the spatial world matter? *Developmental Science, 14*, 1417–1430. http://dx.doi.org/10.1111/j.1467-7687.2011.01088.x

Putnam, S. P., Helbig, A. L., Gartstein, M. A., Rothbard, M. K., & Leerkes, E. (2014). Development and assessment of short and very short forms of the Infant Behavior Questionnaire-Revised. *Journal of Personality Assessment, 96*, 445–458. http://dx.doi.org/10.1080/00223891.2013.841171

Qian, A., Tao, J., Want, X., Liu, H., Ji, L., Yang, C., Ye, Q., Chen, C., Li, J., Cheng, J., Wang, M., & Zhao, K. (2018). Effects of the 2-repeat allele of the DRD4 gene on neural networks associated with the prefrontal cortex in children with ADHD. *Frontiers in Human Neuroscience.* http://dx.doi.org/10.3389/fnhum.2018.00279

Ramirez, N. F., Ramirez, R. R., Clarke, M., Taulu, S., & Kuhl, P. K. (2017). Speech discrimination in 11-month-old bilingual and monolingual infants: A magnetoencephalography study. *Developmental Science, 20*, e12427. http://dx.doi.org/10.1111/desc.12427

Rideout, V. J., & Hamel, E. (2006). *The media family: Electronic media in the lives of infants, toddlers, preschoolers, and their parents.* Kaiser Family Foundation.

Rohner, R.P. & Lansford, J.E. (2017), Deep structure of the human affectional system: Introduction to Interpersonal Acceptance–Rejection Theory. *Journal of Family Theory & Review, 9*, 426–440. https://doi.org/10.1111/jftr.12219

Rothbart, M. K. (2012). Advances in temperament: History, concepts, and measures. In M. Zentner & R. Shiner (Eds.), *Handbook of temperament* (pp. 3–20). Guilford.

Rovee-Collier, C., & Cuevas, K. (2009). The development of infant memory. In M. L. Courage & N. Cowan (Eds.), *The development of memory in infancy and childhood* (2nd ed., pp. 11–41). Psychology Press.

Sagi, A., & Hoffman, M. L. (1976). Empathetic distress in the newborn. *Developmental Psychology, 12*, 175–176.

Sann, C., & Streri, A. (2008). The limits of newborn's grasping to detect texture in a cross-modal transfer task. *Infant Behavior and Development, 31*, 523–531. https://doi.org/10.1016/j.infbeh.2008.03.001

Satterfield-Nash, A., Kotzky, K., Allen, J., Bertolli, J., Moore, C. A., Pereira, I. O., Pessoa, A., Melo, F., Faria e Silva Santelli, A. C., Boyle, C. A., & Peacock, G. (2017). Health and development at age 19–24 months of 19 children who were born with microcephaly and laboratory evidence of congenital Zika virus infection during the 2015 Zika virus outbreak—Brazil, 2017. *Morbidity and Mortality Weekly Report, 66*(49), 1347–1351. http://dx.doi.org/10.15585/mmwr.mm6649a2

Schmitow, C., & Stenberg, G. (2013). Social referencing in 10-month-old infants. *European Journal of Developmental Psychology, 10*, 533–545. http://dx.doi.org/10.1080/17405629.2013.763473

Seavey, C. A, Katz, P. A., & Zalk, S. R. (1975). Baby X: The effect of gender labels on adult responses to infants. *Sex Roles, 1,* 103–109. http://dx.doi.org/10.1007/BF00288004

Shaw, B. A., Krause, N., Chatters, L. M., Connell, C. M., & Ingersoll-Dayton, B. (2004). Emotional support from parents early in life, aging, and health. *Psychology and Aging, 19,* 4–12. http://dx.doi.org/10.1037/0882-7974.19.1.4

Shostak, M. (1981). *Nissa: The life and words of* a !Kung woman. Harvard University Press.

Sidorowicz, L. S., & Lunney, G. S. (1980). Baby X revisited. *Sex Roles, 6,* 67–73. http://dx.doi.org/10.1007/BF00288362

Simion, F., & Giorgio, E. D. (2015). Face perception and processing in early infancy: Inborn predispositions and developmental changes. *Frontiers in Psychology, 6,* 969. http://dx.doi.org/10.3389/fpsyg.2015.00969

Song, L., Tamis-LeMonda, C. S., Yoshikawa, H., Kahana-Kalman, R., & Wu, I. (2012). Language experiences and vocabulary development in Dominican and Mexican infants across the first 2 years. *Developmental Psychology, 48,* 1106–1123. http://dx.doi.org/10.1037/a0026401

Sroufe, L. A. (2017). Attachment theory: A humanistic approach for research and practice across cultures. In S. Gojman-de-Millan, C. Herreman & L. A. Sroufe (Eds.), *Attachment across clinical and cultural perspectives: A relational psychoanalytic approach* (pp. 3–29). Taylor & Francis Group. http://dx.doi.org/10.4324/9781315658100

Stenberg, G. (2017). Does contingency in adults' responding influence 12-month-old infants' social referencing? *Infant Behavior and Development, 49,* 9–20. http://dx.doi.org/10.1016/j.infbeh.2017.06.003

Stovall-McClough, K. C., & Dozier, M. (2004). Forming attachments in foster care: Infant attachment behaviors during the first two months of placement. *Development and Psychopathology, 16,* 253–271. http://dx.doi.org/10.1017/S0954579404044505

Strouse, G. A., & Samson, J. E. (2021). Learning from video: A meta-analysis of the video deficit in children ages 0 to 6 years. *Child Development, 92*(1), e20–e38. http://dx.doi.org/10.1111/cdev.13429

Suir, I., Boonzaaijer, M., Nijmolen, P., Westers, P., & Nuysink, J. (2019). Cross-cultural validity: Canadian norm values of the Alberta Infant Motor Scale evaluated for Dutch infants. *Pediatric Physical Therapy, 31,* 354–358. https://doi.org/10.1097/PEP.0000000000000637

Sulpizio, S., Doi, H., Bornstein, M. H., Cui, J., Esposito, G., & Shinohara, K. (2018). fNIRS reveals enhanced brain activation to female (versus male) infant directed speech (relative to adult directed speech) in young human infants. *Infant Behavior and Development, 52,* 89–96. http://dx.doi.org/10.1016/j.infbeh.2018.05.009

Tamis-LeMonda, C. S., & Bornstein, M. H. (1990). Language, play, and attention at one year. *Infant Behavior & Development, 13,* 85–98. http://dx.doi.org/10.1016/0163-6383(90)90007-U

Tamis-LeMonda, C. S., & Bornstein, M. H. (1994). Specificity in mother-toddler language-play relations across the second year. *Developmental Psychology, 30,* 283–292. http://dx.doi.org/10.1037//0012-1649.30.2.283

Tamis-LeMonda, C. S., & Kahana-Kalman, R. (2009). Mothers' views at the transition to a new baby: Variation across ethnic groups. *Parenting: Science and Practice, 9*, 36–55. http://dx.doi.org/10.1080/15295190802656745

Tanner, J. M. (1962). *Growth at adolescence*. Blackwell Scientific.

Templin, M. C. (1957). *Certain language skills in children: Their development and interrelationships*. University of Minnesota Press.

Travis, K. E., Leonard, M. K., Brown, T. T., Hagler, D. J., Curran, M., Dale, A. M., et al. (2011). Spatiotemporal neural dynamics of word understanding in 12- to 18-month-old infants. *Cerebral Cortex, 21*, 1832–1839. http://dx.doi.org/10.1093/cercor/bhq259

Van de Vondervoort, J. W., & Hamlin, J. K. (2018). The early emergence of sociomoral evaluation: Infants prefer prosocial others. *Current Opinion in Psychology, 20*, 77–81. http://dx.doi.org/10.1016/j.copsyc.2017.08.014

Van IJzendoorn, M. H., & Sagi-Schwartz, A. (2008). Cross-cultural patterns of attachment: Universal and contextual dimensions. In J. Cassidy & P. R. Shaver (Eds.), *Handbook of attachment: Theory, research, and clinical applications* (2nd ed., pp. 880–905). Guilford Press.

Viholainen, H., Ahonen, T., Cantell, M., Lyytinen, P., Lyytinen, H., et al. (2002). Development of early motor skills and language in children at risk for familial dyslexia. *Developmental Medicine & Child Neurology, 44*, 761–769. http://dx.doi.org/10.1111/j.1469-8749.2002.tb00283.x

Viholainen, H., Ahonen, T., Lyytinen, P., Cantell, M., Tolvanen, A., Lyytinen, H. (2006). Early motor development and later language and reading skills in children at risk of familial dyslexia. *Developmental Medicine & Child Neurology, 48*, 367–373. http://dx.doi.org/10.1017/S001216220600079X

Vygotsky, L. S. (1934/1962). *Thought and language*. MIT Press.

Wachs, T. D. (2015). Assessing bioecological influences. In M. H. Bornstein, T. Levanthal, & R. M. Lerner (Eds.), *Handbook of child psychology and developmental science: Ecological settings and processes* (7th ed., vol. 4, pp. 811–846). Wiley.

Wallace, D. B., Franklin, M. B., & Keegan, R. T. (1994). The observing eye: A century of baby diaries. *Human Development, 37*, 1–29.

Waters, E. (1978). The reliability and stability of individual differences in infant-mother attachment. *Child Development, 49*, 483–494. http://dx.doi.org/10.2307/1128714

Watson, J. B. (1924). *Behaviorism*. Norton.

Wheeler, A. C. (2018). Development of infants with congenital Zika syndrome: What do we know and what can we expect? *Pediatrics, 141*(2), 154–160. http://dx.doi.org/10.1542/peds.2017-2038D

Williams, S. T., Mastergeorge, A. M., & Ontai, L. L. (2010). Caregiver involvement in infant peer interactions: Scaffolding in a social context. *Early Childhood Research Quarterly, 25*, 251–266. http://dx.doi.org/10.1016/j.ecresq.2009.11.004

Williams, S. T., Ontai, L. L., & Mastergeorge, A. M. (2007). Reformulating infant and toddler social competence with peers. *Infant Behavior and Development, 30*, 353–365. http://dx.doi.org/10.1016/j.infbeh.2006.10.008

Wilson, E. (1948). *Triple thinkers: Twelve essays on literary subjects*. Oxford University Press.

Yang, Z., Wang, M., Zhu, Z., & Liu, Y. (2020). Coronavirus disease 2019 (COVID-19) and pregnancy: A systematic review. *The Journal of Maternal-Fetal & Neonatal Medicine*, 1–4. http://dx.doi.org/10.1080/14767058.2020.1759541

Yu, J. J., & Gamble, W. C. (2008). Pathways of influence: Marital relationships and their association with parenting styles and sibling relationship quality. *Journal of Child and Family Studies, 17*, 757–778. http://dx.doi.org/10.1007/s10826-008-9188-z

Zeng, L., Xia, S., Yuan, W., Yan, K., Xiao, F., Shao, J., & Zhou, W. (2020). Neonatal early-onset infection with SARS-CoV-2 in 33 neonates born to mothers with COVID-19 in Wuhan, China. *JAMA Pediatrics, 174*, 722–725. http://dx.doi.org/10.1001/jamapediatrics.2020.0878

GLOSSARY

Accommodation: the modification of an existing scheme to apply to a new situation

Acculturating: the process of adopting the customs and beliefs of a new culture

Adaptation: the process whereby schemes are altered by experience; involves two complementary processes: assimilation and accommodation

Affiliative behavior system: social behaviors that cue a desire to interact, including smiling and vocalizing

Altricial: species that are helpless at birth

Anoxia: oxygen deprivation

APGAR: a test administered to newborns to document normal functioning and determine the need for intervention on each of five dimensions: Appearance, Pulse, Grimace, Activity, and Respiration

Arborization: in reference to dendrites, the growth of spines connecting to neighboring cells

Assimilation: processing information according to an existing scheme

Attachment behavior system: controls or coordinates infant activities related to attaining and maintaining proximity to or contact with attachment figures

Attachments: specific, enduring emotional bonds whose existence is of major importance in development; infants' first social relationships, often with parents

Autonomic Nervous System (ANS): an involuntary control system that operates at the level below consciousness and is responsible for heart rate, respiration, digestion, and other basic processes necessary for survival

Axon: the part of the neuron that transmits activity away from the cell body toward other neurons

Baby biography: a psychological diary of the growth of a single child

Bioecological Systems Theory: the nested set of systems of proximal to distal influences over child development

Brightness: luminance

Canalization: the persistence of a developmental outcome despite less than optimal circumstances

Categorical perception: the propensity to treat as similar otherwise discriminable stimuli

Categories of hue: qualitative organization of the color spectrum (as red is distinct from blue)

Cell body: component of the neuron containing the nucleus

Central Nervous System (CNS): the brain and the spinal cord which play a fundamental role in the control of all behavior

Cephalocaudal: a direction of development that means literally from head to tail; development starts at the head and moves down the body

Cesarean section: a surgical procedure involving cutting into the uterus to remove the baby

Chromosomes: contain genes that are composed of chemical codes of DNA that guide development of structure and function

Classical conditioning: a type of learned association

Cognition: all forms of knowing and awareness, including perception, thinking, memory, and decision-making

Confounded (or confound): a factor that cannot be independently tested or isolated, such as the role of genes versus the environment for infants growing up with their biological families

Congenital: applies to structures or functions that are present at the time of birth but are not acquired by heredity

Continuity: consistency in average group scores on some aspect of development over time

Corpus callosum: a bundle of neural fibers that allows communication between the two cortical hemispheres

Cortex: outermost layer of tissue in the brain

Cortical association areas: areas of the brain involved in higher-level processes such as awareness, attention, memory, and the integration of information

Dendrites: part of the neuron that conducts information to the cell body

Didactic caregiving: how parents facilitate infants' understanding of the world around them, including directing attention to objects and events, interpreting external events, and providing opportunities to learn

Directionality: a general principle of physical growth, examples include cephalocaudal and proximodistal

Discriminating sociability: around 2 months of age, infants prefer certain people over others

Disorganized attachment: a type of attachment characterized by contradictory behavior patterns, wherein infants make incomplete movements toward objects or their parents and appear confused or apprehensive about approaching their parents

Down syndrome: a genetic birth disorder associated with intellectual disability

Effectance: behavior can affect the behavior of others in a consistent and predictable fashion

Electrocardiogram: noninvasive electrical technique to measure cardiac function

Embryo: the developing organism from approximately 2 weeks to 8 weeks prenatally

Emotional contagion: when one spontaneously resonates with another's salient emotional expressions, most often observed in response to another's distress

Endogenous: naturally occurring forces internal to the child, such as how the circadian rhythm responds to light-dark cycles

Entrained: biological rhythms that are modified by environmental conditions, such as sleep/wake cycles that fluctuate based on light/darkness patterns

Ethology: the scientific study of animal behavior, often making cross-species comparisons

Exclusivity constraint: a given object has only one name, at least for children learning only one language

Exploratory behavior system: mediates contact with the physical or nonsocial environment

Expressive: children with early vocabularies populated with social formulae and routines, including pronouns and action words

Extrapyramidal system: controls posture and coordination

Fear/Wariness behavior system: coordinates avoidant, wary, or fearful responses to strangers

Fetal alcohol spectrum disorder (FASD): a broad category of birth defects due to maternal alcohol use; considered to be the leading cause of mental and growth retardation with known etiology

Fetus: the developing organism from approximately 8 to 40 weeks prenatally

Figural coherence: the perceptual grouping of elements having an invariant set of spatial relations; example is a point-light display of a person walking

Frontal lobe: a region of the cortex that governs higher-order cognition and voluntary activity

Gametes: reproductive cells: sperm from men and ova from women

Gaze following: when an infant looks in a new location based on the gaze (and sometimes head movement) of another person

Genes: contain the chemical codes of DNA

Genotype: the genetic makeup of the individual

Gesture: nonverbal supports to communication and language, such as pointing

Goodness-of-fit: match between the child and the developmental context

Gyrus: bumps or ridges on the cerebral cortex

Habituation: the process whereby infants become bored with the stimulus, suggesting they recognize it as the same as seen previously, and their level of attention declines

Hemispheres: the two halves of the brain

Hue: what is typically thought of as color based on the wavelength of light

Independence of systems: components that are differentially developed at a given time and develop along different trajectories

Indiscriminately sociable: in the first 2 months of life, infants interact with people but prefer no particular person

Individual differences: how organisms differ from each other, resulting from their unique combination of biology and experience

Induction: using a limited set of examples to draw conclusions that permit inferences about new cases

Infant-directed speech: speech used with infants; simplifies adult speech in that it has higher pitch, exaggerated intonation, sing-song rhythm, abbreviated utterances, and repetition

Innate: present at birth or biologically programmed to develop at a particular time

Insecure-avoidant attachment: a type of attachment in which infants appear unconcerned by their parents' absence and actively avoid interaction when reuniting with their parents

Insecure-resistant attachment: a type of attachment in which infants are unable to use their parents as a secure base to explore; although they are distressed by their parents' departure, they behave ambivalently on reunion or seek contact but angrily reject the parent

Interiorization: making the external world accessible to the internal mind

Internal working model: a schema of how relationships work based on early parent-child-environment interactions

Joint attention: when two people, such as an infant and adult, attend to an object or event at the same time

Labor: involuntary uterine contractions, beginning at the top of the muscle, that literally force the fetus out of the uterus

Limbic system: structures in the brain that support emotion and memory

Material caregiving: the manner in which parents structure infants' physical environments, including provision of toys and books and restrictions on physical freedom

Maternal gatekeeping: activities that mothers engage in to limit others', particularly fathers', interactions with their children

Myelin sheath: a fatty layer of the neuron that insulates the axon and facilitates the speed of information transmission

Natural experiment: a study using naturally occurring groupings of participants instead of assigning participants to different treatment conditions, such as children reared in an orphanage compared to children reared by their parents

Neuron: core component of the nervous system composed of a cell body, nucleus, axon, and dendrites

Neurotransmitters: neurochemicals which neurons use to communicate with each other

Nominal insight: the realization that things have names

Nonshared environment: environmental differences that act on individuals in the same situation or setting differently

Norm: the average for a population

Novelty responsiveness: following habitation, the amount infants' look at a novel stimulus relative to a familiar one

Nucleus: central part of the neuron that contains DNA

Nurturant caregiving: providing infants' basic survival needs for protection, supervision, and sustenance

Occipital lobe: region of the cortex that governs the processing of visual information

Operant conditioning: learning that involves associations between actions and their consequences

Oxytocin: a hormone secreted by the pituitary gland which induces contractions and then labor; also plays a role in regulation of social behavior

Parietal lobe: region of the cortex that governs the processing of temperature, taste, touch, and directs motor movements

Phenotype: the observed characteristics of the individual

Phonology: sounds that are linguistically meaningful in the language

Physical caregiving: promoting infants' physical development, such as providing toys and activities to foster development of fine and gross motor skills

Pragmatics: the social rules that dictate everyday usage of language

Proximodistal: a direction of development that means literally from close to far; development starts at the center of the body and moves to the extremities

Pyramidal system: controls precise, rapid, and skilled movements of the extremities

Quickening: felt movement of fetus *in utero*, beginning around 4 months

Referential: children with early vocabularies that consist of a high proportion of object labels and whose speech provides concrete information

Reflexes: integrated and organized automatic stimulus-response behaviors

Reliable: a measure that can be used by multiple observers or across multiple assessments to obtain the same score or outcome

Representational thinking: the ability to think about people and objects in their absence

Reticular formation: a subcortical structure that regulates sleep/wake patterns

Saturation: color vividness

Secure attachment: a type of attachment in which infants use their parents as a secure base from which they confidently engage with other people and explore the physical environment

Secure base: an attachment figure, such as a parent, who provides infants with confidence to explore unfamiliar people or aspects of their environment

Self-concept: how we perceive, evaluate, or think about ourselves

Semantics: the meaning of words and phrases

Sensitive parenting: nurturant, attentive, responsive, nonrestrictive parental care

Social caregiving: efforts to involve infants in interpersonal exchanges, including soothing, touching, smiling, and vocalizing

Social cognition: the ways to perceive and understand social interaction, the people with whom we interact, and differences between others' perspectives and knowledge and our own

Social referencing: the deliberate search for information from other people to help clarify uncertain or ambiguous events

Somatic nervous system: voluntary control of body movements via skeletal muscles

Specificity principle: specific experiences at specific times shape specific developmental outcomes in specific people in specific ways

Stability: consistency over time in the relative ranking of individuals in a group

Still-face paradigm: an experimental protocol that has an adult, typically the mother, cease responding to the social bids of the infant which normally disrupts interaction

Strange situation: an experimental protocol to study attachment that is designed to expose infants to stress to observe attachment behaviors

Stranger anxiety: when infants react negatively to unfamiliar adults

Sudden Infant Death Syndrome (SIDS): the unexpected and unexplained death of an infant younger than 1 year of age

Sulcus: a groove or indentation on the cerebral cortex

Symbols: something or someone that stands for or suggests another entity

Synapses: connections between axons and dendrites which serve communication between neurons

Syntax: grammar or the rules for combining words into meaningful communications

Taxonomic constraint: the tendency to interpret new words as referring, not only to the object seen and labeled with a word, but to other objects of the same kind

Temperament: the biologically based source of stable individual differences in behavioral functioning

Temporal lobe: region of the cortex that governs the processing of auditory information and language comprehension and production

Teratogens: environmental factors harmful to the fetus

Theory of mind: the understanding that mental states, including beliefs, intents, desires, pretending, and knowledge, guide behavior

Transactional principle: the reciprocity of mutual influences of organism (e.g., child) and organism (e.g., parent), or organism and environment, over time

Trimester: a three-month division of pregnancy

Trisomy-21: a genetic disorder resulting from having an extra chromosome, also known as Down syndrome

Trust: the idea that someone can be counted on to respond when signaled

Turn taking: the alternation of speakers in normal conversation or interaction

Užgiris-Hunt Ordinal Scales of Psychological Development: criterion-based test that assesses infant performance on Piagetian-based tasks

Valid: a test or assessment that measures what we think it measures

Viewpoint invariance: the understanding that an object viewed from different perspectives is the same object

Visual acuity: the degree of resolution of detail

Visual cliff: an experimental technique used to measure infant depth perception

Zygote: the developing organism from conception to 2 weeks prenatally

AUTHOR INDEX

Note: *Italic* page numbers refer to figures.

SUBJECT INDEX

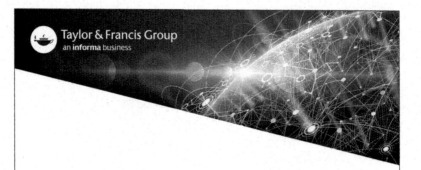